Pregnancy Loss

A guide to what complementary and alternative medicine can offer

JANETTA BENSOUILAH

Traditional Acupuncturist
CAM Practitioner in private practice
Surrey, UK

Radcliffe Publishing
London • New York

Radcliffe Publishing Ltd
33–41 Dallington Street
London
EC1V 0BB
United Kingdom

www.radcliffepublishing.com
Electronic catalogue and worldwide online ordering facility.

British Library Cataloguing in Publication Data

A catalogue record for this book is available from the British Library.

ISBN-13: 978 184619 374 3

The paper used for the text pages of this book is FSC® certified. FSC (The Forest Stewardship Council®) is an international network to promote responsible management of the world's forests.

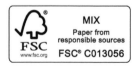

MIX
Paper from
responsible sources
FSC® C013056

Typeset by Pindar NZ, Auckland, New Zealand
Printed and bound by TJI Digital, Padstow, Cornwall, UK

Contents

Preface

Professionally I am an outsider to mainstream medicine, but in almost two decades of working closely with women I have obtained a clear understanding of the frustrations, difficulties and deep sadness that patients and health professionals alike often experience when a pregnancy is lost. Over the years I have practised a range of traditional therapies, and have seen the profound benefits that women experience when care is offered with a freedom to focus on the individual that is sometimes not possible within the environment of conventional medicine. Wonderful things can be achieved with modern medicine, and at its best it can offer tremendous support and sometimes hope to women who find themselves facing a threatened or failing pregnancy, or in the terrible aftermath of a lost one. However, this is not always the case, and sadly women do on occasion feel uncared for or brushed aside by medical professionals, especially when their loss occurs early in pregnancy.

In an age of almost inexhaustible information where modern medicine offers the promise of remarkable management of many illnesses, it can be deeply shocking for a woman to discover that her miscarriage is regarded as a medical non-event. Worse still, she will have to experience at least another loss and probably two more before her doctor will initiate investigations. Many women seek answers outside medicine and will go to enormous lengths and try almost anything to prevent such a loss happening again. Some will be taken in by irresponsible appeals to desperate patients by practitioners of all kinds of therapies in the largely unregulated world of complementary and alternative medicine (CAM). CAM is a broad term which has come to embrace many therapeutic disciplines. There has been much progress in recent years in improving the educational standards of many of these, and their professionalisation continues to march on. However, the lack of formal or statutory regulation of much of what constitutes CAM presents a somewhat confusing picture for those working outside it. This can lead to unwillingness among some involved in conventional medicine to actively engage in the field, despite its ongoing increasing use by the public, a high self-referral rate by those who have the means to access CAM, and a growing evidence base. Tensions continue to exist between conventional medicine and CAM, and perhaps they always will on some level. My hope is that this book will contribute to developing a sound knowledge of the different perspectives within the context of pregnancy loss. Healthcare professionals may not actively administer any of the therapies that come under the CAM umbrella (although increasing numbers of doctors, midwives and nurses do so), but a knowledge of what women may gain from these therapies will help to ensure that mutual respect for the practices of others is shown. This book aims to contribute to this process.

Through my clinical work as an independent practitioner of complementary medicine, I have gained many insights into the remarkable resilience of women who have shared with me their experiences of pregnancy loss in all its forms, from early miscarriage right through to the dreadful shock of stillbirth. The purpose of the book is to help any healthcare professional, like myself, who comes into close contact with women in these circumstances and who wishes to gain greater awareness of both the medical aspects of pregnancy loss and how the implementation of sound and professional CAM may contribute to the lives of those affected. The book contains occasional insights from my clinical work in the form of real-life accounts of my patients (in the usual tradition, their names and distinguishing details have been changed in order to protect their privacy). The rationale for including these has been to illustrate a thought or a salient aspect of whatever is under discussion.

Throughout the text, for reasons of brevity I have often used the terms 'parents' or 'couples' when referring to bereaved mothers and their partners, although I recognise that some women may not have a partner, or may have a female partner who is affected by the loss. I have endeavoured to adhere to UK definitions of loss, and only use the phrase 'miscarriage' to refer to losses before 24 weeks. Where I use the phrase 'pregnancy loss' this covers loss at any gestational stage. If errors occur here, I hope that the overall sense is conveyed sufficiently clearly to allow these minor slips to be overlooked. I am aware that I have taken a general approach to the whole field of CAM rather than emphasising the many differences between the vast range of disciplines. I sincerely hope that the end result is not an oversimplification of the complexities of each discipline. I have also tried to avoid using unintelligible jargon for what may be a wide readership with little awareness of the language used in each therapy, and have opted instead to whet the appetite for further exploration by those who wish to know more.

My main priority has been to present in one text a basis for practitioners of many disciplines, including those in mainstream medicine, to be able to work knowledgeably and confidently with women who have experienced pregnancy loss who may be either using or hoping to use CAM. It is my profound belief that those in the field of CAM have much to offer these women, and I hope that this book stimulates other professionals to make a rigorous contribution to assisting women in their healing, comfort and care in the aftermath, recovery from and prevention of pregnancy loss.

Janetta Bensouilah
February 2011

About the author

Janetta Bensouilah holds qualifications in several traditional disciplines, including acupuncture, aromatherapy and reflexology, and has an MSc in Chinese herbal medicine. Her final thesis explored in depth the use of Chinese herbal medicine in modern gynaecology treatments. She has been in practice for almost two decades, and over the years the many strands to her work have included writing and teaching several professional-level complementary and alternative medicine courses both in the UK and overseas. First and foremost a practitioner, Janetta now focuses on working with women using acupuncture and herbal medicine in her private practice in Surrey, England.

Acknowledgements

I offer heartfelt thanks to all my patients who time and time again have shown me how complementary and alternative medicine helps people to overcome tremendous difficulties and gain improved health and well-being. I have learned a great deal from the feelings and memories that they have shared with me, some of which appear here, and I am truly grateful for the opportunity that they have given me to develop and learn. Every day of my working life I am inspired by all of these women. Over almost two decades in practice and teaching, I have been fortunate to have the support of many friends and colleagues who have helped me to mature both personally and professionally. I offer my thanks to each and every one of them. A final but very important thank you to my family, especially Michel, for his love, support and enduring patience throughout all the times I have disappeared, taking Jasmine and Rosie with me for their quiet inspiring company sitting by my feet during the long hours at the computer.

CHAPTER 1

Pregnancy loss defined

INTRODUCTION

An early miscarriage may be a normal, natural way to end an unhealthy pregnancy, or it may not. It might be an event which indicates disorder that can be corrected or at least managed, thus reducing any threat to future pregnancies. No one knows for certain the exact prevalence of miscarriage. However, it is estimated that around 15% of clinically recognised pregnancies will end in miscarriage, with a further 15–25% of subclinical pregnancies miscarrying before any signs or symptoms of pregnancy develop.[1-3] Nowadays, with advances in pregnancy detection technology, pregnancies can routinely be detected that would have gone unnoticed in earlier times, leading to an apparent increase in the number of miscarriages, with researchers now viewing recurrent miscarriage as far more common than was once assumed to be the case.[4] In addition to loss through miscarriage, pregnancies can be doomed by their very nature, as in the case of ectopic or lethal abnormality of the baby, or in the later stages they may result in stillbirth.

DEFINITIONS AND TERMINOLOGY

The World Health Organization (WHO) has defined miscarriage as the loss of an embryo or fetus weighing 500 grams or less, which corresponds to 20 to 22 weeks' gestation, whereas the legal definition in the UK is the loss of a baby with a gestational age of 24 weeks or less, and in North America it is 20 weeks.[5] After 24 weeks' gestation, spontaneous loss of a baby is termed a stillbirth, but if the baby dies in the womb and is not miscarried it is referred to as an intrauterine death. Although 'abortion' is the correct medical term for any loss of a pregnancy before viability, and 'spontaneous abortion' is sometimes used to refer to miscarriage, there has been a move away from the use of these terms among health professionals. The Royal College of Obstetricians and Gynaecologists suggests that, when talking with parents, the word 'miscarriage' is used, and it is reported that after 14 weeks parents prefer the term 'stillbirth', as this shows an understanding of the meaning of the loss that has been experienced.[6]

Miscarriage
Early, late, missed and spontaneous miscarriages
Spontaneous miscarriage is the most common complication of early pregnancy. Loss of a baby before week 13 of gestation is called an early miscarriage, and the majority of pregnancy losses occur during this period, in fact in the first 8 weeks of pregnancy. If the physical process of miscarriage has not occurred – that is, the uterus has not expelled the failed pregnancy – it is termed a 'missed miscarriage', and it can be particularly distressing for couples to discover at the 12-week scan that the baby had died some time beforehand. Mid-trimester or late miscarriages occur after week 13 of gestation and are relatively rare, affecting less than 3% of all pregnancies.[1] The causes of early and late miscarriage differ considerably, and late miscarriages in particular should always be medically investigated in order to find the underlying cause.

Recurrent miscarriage
Defined as the loss of three or more consecutive pregnancies, recurrent miscarriage (RM) affects around 1–2% of conceptions, and in 50% of these cases no cause can be identified despite major advances in understanding in recent years.[1,5] Some clinicians argue that two miscarriages justify investigation, because the likelihood of finding a cause is more or less the same as after two or three miscarriages. However, although it can be hard for women who have experienced two miscarriages to accept this, undergoing investigations which can be stressful and expensive may not be their best option, as 70–80% of couples who experience RM eventually achieve a successful pregnancy without any medical intervention.[4,5]

Threatened miscarriage

Vaginal bleeding with or without pain in the first 24 weeks of pregnancy is relatively common, with the estimated incidence ranging from 20% to 50% of clinically recognised pregnancies.[3,5] There are several possible causes of bleeding and abdominal pain in pregnancy, including those coincidental to the pregnancy (*see* Box 1.1). As well as bleeding, a diagnosis of threatened miscarriage is reached with the help of an ultrasound scan and an examination showing a closed cervix. Although threatened miscarriages are always alarming, the probability of the pregnancy continuing successfully is high, as 50% of all pregnancies involving bleeding continue. If bleeding occurs at 10 weeks, more than 90% of pregnancies continue, and if it occurs at 13 weeks, more than 99% continue.[5] Furthermore, studies have shown that there is no damage to the baby as a result of the bleeding.[2]

Inevitable miscarriage

If the cervix starts to open, a threatened miscarriage becomes an inevitable one as the cervix cannot close again. The opening of the cervix usually causes cramping pain as the uterus attempts to expel the fetus and the bleeding becomes more severe. If any of the pregnancy tissue remains in the uterus, the miscarriage is termed 'incomplete' and an evacuation of retained products of conception (ERPC) procedure is usually performed, although expectant management may be offered if deemed appropriate by the medical team.

BOX 1.1: Common causes of vaginal bleeding and abdominal pain in pregnancy

Pregnancy-related causes
- Ectopic pregnancy
- Hydatidiform mole
- Miscarriage

Coincidental to pregnancy: gynaecological causes
- Ruptured corpus luteum
- Rupture or torsion of ovarian cyst
- Torsion or degeneration of fibroid

Causes unrelated to pregnancy
- Appendicitis
- Cholecystitis
- Dysfunctional uterine bleeding
- Endometriosis
- Intestinal obstruction
- Pelvic inflammatory disease
- Renal colic

Missed miscarriage

In some cases, when the fetus dies there are no clinical signs of miscarriage as the uterus fails to expel the fetus. This is termed a missed miscarriage, or early fetal demise. In some cases, women can recall a stage in the pregnancy when they noticed changes, usually a lessening or disappearance of nausea or breast tenderness, but this is not always the case, and the shock of discovering that the pregnancy has ended with no apparent warning can be immense. Although the body will usually expel the pregnancy eventually, many women prefer an ERPC to be performed as it formally ends the pregnancy.

Ectopic pregnancy

A pregnancy that occurs outside the uterine cavity is described as ectopic, and most ectopic pregnancies (98%) occur in the Fallopian tube, with the remainder sited on the ovary, in the cervix or in the abdominal cavity. Ectopic pregnancies are fairly common and their incidence is increasing, now affecting approximately one in every 200 pregnancies in the general maternal population. Although the maternal mortality rate associated with ectopic pregnancy has decreased significantly in the last quarter of a century, it remains the leading cause of first-trimester maternal death in western countries.[5] The increase in the numbers of ectopic pregnancies may be due to a number of factors, including higher rates of assisted conception, and greater sensitivity of diagnostic tests leading to earlier detection, whereas in previous times spontaneous resolution might have occurred prior to detection. Another factor accounting for the increase is the higher number of older women who are conceiving. Women aged 35–44 years are three times more likely to have an ectopic pregnancy than women aged 15–24 years.[1]

The presentation of ectopic pregnancy varies considerably, but one of the most common early symptoms is lower abdominal pain with or without bleeding, and a brown vaginal discharge, sometimes developing into heavier bleeding. Severe abdominal pain is a later feature and localisation is not specific. Abdominal pain associated with rupture tends to be much more intense, and there will be accompanying signs of peritonism on abdominal palpation. It is essential that medical care is sought if an ectopic pregnancy is suspected.

Gestational trophoblastic disease and hydatidiform moles

Gestational trophoblastic disease (GTD) is an uncommon cause of first-trimester vaginal bleeding, and encompasses a range of conditions involving abnormal proliferation of gestational trophoblast tissue, the most common one being the usually benign partial hydatidiform mole. Complete and partial moles can occur, the difference being that complete moles may develop into an invasive cancer. Essentially, moles develop from an accident at fertilisation, resulting in either no developing embryo in the case of complete moles, or one with three sets of chromosomes in partial moles, but in both cases the result is rapidly developing placental tissue. Persistent bleeding, nausea and a larger than expected uterus for gestational age accompany the moles, which are detected by ultrasound scan and removed surgically. If pregnancy is more advanced, medical termination may be used instead, and in all cases careful medical follow-up should be arranged.

Preterm labour

Preterm labour (PTL) can be defined as regular uterine contractions that cause dilation of the cervix between 24 and 36 weeks of gestation. It is estimated that around 11% of all pregnancies end in preterm delivery, and the rate is increasing. The latter trend reflects the increasing numbers of multiple pregnancies resulting from infertility treatments,[7] as multiples are particularly prone to delivering early.

Intrauterine death and stillbirth

According to the International Stillbirth Alliance, 4.5 million stillbirths occur each year worldwide, with the rate in developed countries estimated to be one in 100–200 pregnancies.[8] There is no agreed international definition of stillbirth of a baby. The WHO defines it as the death of a baby after

22 weeks of pregnancy, or when the baby weighs at least 500 grams. In the UK it is considered to be the death of a baby after 24 weeks, in Sweden after 28 weeks, in Norway after 16 weeks, and in the USA and Australia after 20 weeks.[8] Intrauterine death refers to the situation where a baby dies in the womb but is not spontaneously miscarried. Medical induction of labour brings about delivery, which is then termed a stillbirth. Multifetal pregnancies are more at risk of intrauterine death than singletons, and the higher the number of fetuses, the greater the risk. A baby of any gestational age who is born demonstrating signs of life, such as breathing, a heartbeat or pulsation of the umbilical cord, is regarded as alive and acquires the same legal status as other humans and is owed a duty of care.[6] Babies who are born at the cusp of viability present enormous difficulties and dilemmas, and a high level of understanding, support and sensitivity is required for all involved.

Selective fetal reduction and multifetal pregnancy reduction

Selective or multifetal pregnancy reduction may be offered in triplet and higher-order multiple pregnancies in order to reduce the risk of preterm labour, intrauterine growth restriction and other morbidities associated with multiple pregnancies. It may also be performed in twin pregnancies where one of the babies is found to have a serious abnormality.

REFERENCES

1 Edmonds DK. *Dewhurst's Textbook of Obstetrics and Gynaecology.* 7th edn. Oxford: Blackwell Publishing; 2007.

2 Scher J, Dix C. *Preventing Miscarriage.* New York: Collins; 2005.

3 Regan L. *Miscarriage: what every woman needs to know.* London: Orion; 2001.

4 Cohen J. *Coming to Term.* New Brunswick, NJ: Rutgers University Press; 2007.

5 James DK, Steer PJ, Weiner CP *et al. High Risk Pregnancy Management Options.* 3rd edn. Philadelphia, PA: Elsevier; 2006.

6 Schott J, Henley A, Kohner N. *Pregnancy Loss and the Death of a Baby: guidelines for professionals.* 3rd edn. London: Sands; 2007.

7 Gilbert E, Harmon J. *Manual of High Risk Pregnancy and Delivery.* 3rd edn. St Louis, MO: Mosby; 2003.

8 www.stillbirthalliance.org

CHAPTER 2

Causes and risk factors

INTRODUCTION

Although there have been major advances in the medical understanding of pregnancy loss over the past couple of decades, much remains unknown, with many possible causes and associations, complicated by different causes operating at different gestational stages. It is also probable that in some cases of pregnancy loss, the presence of dual pathology complicates matters further. A cause is identified in only around 50% of all cases of recurrent miscarriage (RM),[1,2] and for many women the lack of an identifiable cause following investigation can provoke significant emotional disturbance in an age when answers to common medical problems are expected. For some women, the frustration of having to undergo three miscarriages before investigations are undertaken, only to be told that no reason can be found and therefore no treatment is available, can be powerful and damaging. One patient recounted how, after her second miscarriage, she had willed the third pregnancy to proceed to what she believed would be its inevitable premature end so that she could start having tests, a cause could be found and treatment given, and then she might have a better chance of successfully carrying a baby.

Spontaneous miscarriage is the most common complication of pregnancy, and up to 25% of all women are affected by a single, one-off miscarriage, the cause of which will remain unknown. The causes and risk factors that are explored here are all known or suspected to play a part in some cases of miscarriage, but for an individual woman it is unlikely that she will be able to know for sure what led to her spontaneous loss unless specific medical investigations are undertaken, and even then there may not be an answer. In most cases the event is random and unlikely to repeat itself in a future pregnancy. On one level it may seem a harsh reality that the spontaneous loss of a pregnancy is largely down to bad luck, but on the other hand this does mean that there is a good chance that most couples will go on to have a successful pregnancy.

In their desperation to seek answers with regard to their situation, couples who are experiencing pregnancy loss are in a vulnerable position

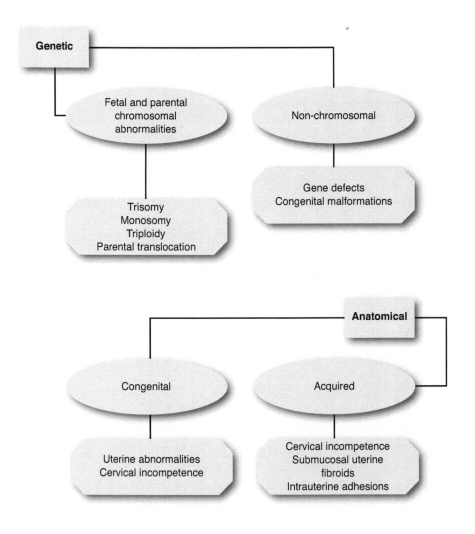

FIGURE 2.1: Genetic and anatomical causes of pregnancy loss.

and may be willing to try any measures, or avoid doing anything, that may affect their pregnancies, whether or not there is any evidence to support such actions. This can have major implications for how they live their day-to-day lives, and for their emotional well-being. It is hoped this chapter will help readers to understand the current state of medical knowledge about the causes of pregnancy loss, which in turn should help them to gain a clearer perspective on any individual case.

The causes of pregnancy loss fall into one or more of the following categories:
➤ genetic
➤ anatomical
➤ hormonal
➤ immunological
➤ thrombophilic
➤ infectious
➤ environmental.

There are several suspected causes, but relatively few that are proven and widely acknowledged. There is considerable ongoing debate about cause and association, as precise mechanisms remain elusive even in known aetiologies. The aim here is to outline the most common possible causes, with an emphasis on discussing those where the evidence is most persuasive. However, it is worth noting that new studies and discoveries are ongoing in this field, and what may be a suspected cause today might be proven or discounted in the future.

GENETIC CAUSES
Chromosomal abnormalities
Chromosomal abnormalities are the most frequent cause of early, spontaneous, isolated miscarriages, but in cases of RM they are a less frequent cause, affecting around 2–4% of cases.[3] Chromosomes are strands of genetic material that contain the genetic code which makes up an individual. A human being has 46 chromosomes in every cell, 23 chromosomes being inherited from each parent. Before conception, the chromosomes of the egg and sperm cells first divide, a process known as *meiosis*, so that each has only 23 chromosomes. Subsequently, at fertilisation, the normal chromosome

number of 46 is restored as a result of the fusion of sperm and egg. Around 12–24 hours after fertilisation, a complex process of vigorous cell division and multiplication, known as *mitosis*, begins. At this stage some chromosomes may be lost or damaged, and if one of the chromosomes is abnormal, or an incorrect number of chromosomes is left in the fertilised egg, an abnormal fetus may develop. The vast majority of such abnormalities are incompatible with life and will miscarry at an early stage, although some will continue to birth and may or may not survive.

Trisomies

Trisomies arise from abnormal meiosis in the egg prior to fertilisation, resulting in fetal cells having three copies of one type of chromosome. Down's syndrome is perhaps the best known trisomy. Although the mechanisms involved are not fully understood, it is known that female hormones control meiosis and that with declining egg numbers, chromosomal separation becomes less effective. Therefore trisomies are much more common in older mothers. However, focusing on female age alone reveals only part of the picture, as it is specifically how close the woman is to menopause in terms of decreasing egg supply that affects the degree of chaos of meiotic events.[4] For example, it is known that some RM women start forming recurrent trisomies in their mid-thirties.[2] If one miscarriage is experienced, there is a slightly increased risk of having further losses due to a trisomy, and if this is the known cause of a previous miscarriage, the woman will be advised to undergo testing in any subsequent pregnancy. Although maternal age is undoubtedly a major contributory factor in terms of chromosomal causes of pregnancy loss, the effect of paternal age is less clear, with conflicting findings in the literature.[5–7]

Monosomy

Monosomies occur when one chromosome is missing, and they account for around 15% of miscarriages. The commonest type of monosomy is found in girls and results in Turner's syndrome.

Triploidy

When an embryo contains an extra set of chromosomes, this is called a triploidy. It may result from the egg being fertilised by more than one sperm; maternal age is not a factor here. Some will miscarry very early, whereas others progress and are accompanied by placental abnormalities and do not survive to birth. A partial hydatidiform mole is an example of a triploidy. It contains an embryo or fetus with three sets of chromosomes.

Parental translocations

In 0.3% of cases of spontaneous miscarriage and 3–5% of cases of recurrent miscarriage the cause is parental translocation.[8–10] This condition affects one or more rarely both parents, and occurs when a piece of one chromosome breaks off and attaches to another chromosome. In a balanced translocation there is no loss or gain of important genetic material and the person is asymptomatic. However, when they produce eggs or sperm and the cells divide, they only receive half the parental chromosomes. When the individual tries to have children, if fertilisation occurs with one of the abnormal eggs or sperm the embryo will inherit the translocation and either will be a balanced carrier and compatible with normal life, or will be unbalanced and either miscarry or produce abnormalities. Both males and females can be carriers of translocations. There is some evidence that paternal translocations may have less impact on reproductive outcome than those carried by women.[2] Even if a couple have had a healthy child, followed by subsequent miscarriages, it is possible that the baby inherited the balanced translocation and therefore survived, but the miscarried babies were chromosomally abnormal. Generally the outlook is positive for balanced translocations, eventually resulting in healthy offspring, and parents with identifiable chromosomal abnormalities should be referred to genetic counsellors for guidance.

Non-chromosomal genetic problems

Gene defects

Genetics research and knowledge are expanding rapidly and there is much work being done on the effects of gene defects on all aspects of human disease. It is very likely that in the future many gene defects will be identified as causing sporadic and recurrent miscarriages. Some of the known causes under discussion in this chapter are genetically driven (e.g. genetic thrombophilic mutations, certain neural tube defects and some immunological causes).

Congenital malformations

In congenital malformations the baby has a structural or functional defect or malformation. Some of the most familiar ones are the neural tube defects *spina bifida, encephalocoele* and *anencephaly.* Spina bifida has a strong genetic association, but it is exaggerated when an environmental factor such as a deficiency in folic acid intake coexists. Up to 40% of neural tube defects are miscarried, and they account for around 5% of spontaneous miscarriages.[8]

What causes chromosomal, genetic and congenital defects?

The causes of most of these abnormalities remain unknown, but the following factors are either known to be involved or have been suggested by some research findings:

➤ maternal age
➤ paternal age
➤ radiation
➤ dietary factors (e.g. maternal intake of folic acid and neural tube defects)
➤ certain drugs (e.g. thalidomide)
➤ infections (e.g. viruses)
➤ maternal or paternal exposure to certain chemicals
➤ uncontrolled diabetes
➤ alcohol abuse.

ANATOMICAL CAUSES

Congenital or acquired abnormalities in the cervix or uterus can cause both early and late miscarriages. In early pregnancy the embryo may be unable to implant properly, and in later pregnancy the development of the baby may be restricted by the presence of the anatomical problems. The link between some congenital uterine anomalies and RM has been established, leading to suggestions that treatment may result in an improved pregnancy outcome.[11] However, it is worth noting that anatomical abnormalities are very common, and it is possible that the majority of women with uterine abnormalities will not experience any serious obstetric problems.

Congenital abnormalities

Congenital uterine malformations that are not uncommon include complete or partial septate uterine development, the bicornuate or 'heart-shaped' uterus, and the more extreme complete duplication of the uterus and cervix, known as uterus didelphys. These are associated with:

➤ late miscarriage
➤ preterm delivery
➤ spontaneous early miscarriage
➤ ectopic pregnancy
➤ fetal malpresentation
➤ a higher than average Caesarean delivery rate.[10]

However, it is notable that quite major anomalies have little if any impact in some women, and it is not known to what extent these anomalies contribute to overall pregnancy loss. The higher prevalence of uterine abnormalities in women with late miscarriage and preterm delivery may reflect a concurrent problem of cervical incompetence.

Cervical incompetence

Also termed cervical insufficiency, cervical incompetence is well recognised as a potential cause of mid-trimester miscarriage, and although some cases involve mechanical weakness, in the majority of cases there is normal cervical anatomy, but evidence of subclinical intrauterine infection. However, whether infection is the result or cause of premature cervical dilation remains unknown.[10] In addition to being a congenital problem, cervical incompetence may follow mechanical trauma such as excessive dilation at the time of curettage, cervical biopsy or occasionally a difficult vaginal delivery. Preterm labour (PTL) has been linked to cervical incompetence in single and multiple pregnancies. In the case of the latter, the risk is higher, and as PTL is the major cause of neonatal death in multiple pregnancies, cervical screening is useful for identifying those at risk, although there is uncertainty as to whether the standard treatment of inserting a stitch (cerclage) improves pregnancy outcome.[12,13]

Acquired abnormalities

Submucosal uterine fibroids can present problems in both early and late pregnancy. Implantation may be adversely affected in the early days of pregnancy, and as the baby develops, the size, shape or location of the fibroid may affect placentation, prevent the baby from developing fully and result in late miscarriage or premature labour. Intrauterine adhesions (Asherman's syndrome) are an acquired abnormality associated with RM, and can result from trauma after ERPC or endometrial curettage, or an episode of endometritis. The resultant fibrosis, decreased uterine cavity volume, endometrial inflammation and abnormal placentation are thought to be the causes of pregnancy loss, although the exact causal relationships remain unclear.[10]

HORMONAL CAUSES

It has long been thought that many cases of miscarriage are secondary to an underlying endocrine imbalance, but the evidence for a clear causal link remains elusive. *Luteal phase deficiency* has traditionally been the focus of research in this area, and refers to insufficient progesterone secretion by the corpus luteum, resulting in inadequate preparation of the endometrium for implantation and a subsequent failure to maintain early pregnancy. However, studies have shown that there are similarities between luteal phase progesterone profiles and endometrial biopsy findings in both successful pregnancies and those that are lost.[12] In cases of sporadic miscarriage with luteal phase deficiency, it is not likely to be repeated, and there is no convincing evidence that treatment of the luteal phase defect improves pregnancy outcome.[10]

Women who experience RM have a higher incidence of polycystic ovaries than the general population, but the exact relationships between this finding, polycystic ovary syndrome (PCOS) and pregnancy loss are still under discussion. It used to be thought that hypersecretion of luteinising hormone was the culprit, but this theory has now been discounted as further studies have shown suppression of this to be ineffective. However, the insulin resistance, obesity and hyperandrogenaemia which are also features of the syndrome are all factors associated with miscarriage. Administration of the insulin-sensitising agent metformin is believed to improve endometrial receptivity and implantation, and has been shown to reduce the risk of miscarriage in patients with PCOS.[14]

Although it was once believed that thyroid dysfunction and diabetes mellitus predisposed a woman to miscarriage, it is now known that once these conditions have been recognised and treated, there is no greater risk of miscarriage than in the general population, and subclinical cases are not thought to be causative. However, if left untreated or poorly controlled, both conditions are associated with infertility and miscarriage.

IMMUNOLOGICAL CAUSES

Despite advances in understanding of the immunological disruption to pregnancy that can occur in some women, and the availability of treatments that might address some of these conditions, the precise role of the immune system in pregnancy loss remains uncertain. For a pregnancy to be successful, complex adaptations in the immune response need to occur so that the maternal reaction to the embryo, which is essentially 50% foreign tissue, is life-sustaining rather than lethal. Whereas pregnancy was once viewed as a conflict between fetus and maternal immunity, a conceptual reframing has been taking place, and the many cooperative interactions between the two are now emphasised in reproductive immunology.[15] When responses go awry, two immunological mechanisms are involved, namely those involving autoimmune factors and alloimmunity.

Alloimmune factors

Simply defined as immunity against foreign substances, one of the most miraculous aspects of human pregnancy is that in most cases the alloimmune relationship between mother and fetus is able to adapt to a unique position of preventing rejection of the growing fetus. Cells of the immune system found in the uterine wall, known as T cells, produce protective, growth-promoting cytokines that allow the pregnancy to flourish. More specifically, healthy adaptation leads to suppression of the embryotoxic Th1 response and dominance of the pro-pregnancy Th2 response, although exactly how this happens remains unclear. It is known that dominance of the Th1 response in early pregnancy is linked with early RM,[1] but it is an oversimplification to view the highly complex maternal–fetal immune relationship as simply one of tolerance of foreign tissue. Convenient as the Th1/Th2 hypothesis is for explaining pregnancy loss, research continues to produce findings which indicate that this is far from the full picture.

Human leukocyte antigens and natural killer cells

Although uterine natural killer (uNK) cells are thought to play a significant role in the establishment and maintenance of early pregnancy, their precise function remains unknown, and there is much controversy and debate about their role in pregnancy failure. Unsurprisingly, tests and treatments in this area are similarly controversial (*see* Chapter 4).

In a successful pregnancy, human leukocyte antigen G (HLA-G) interacts with fetal tissues and prevents attack by natural killer (NK) cells, allowing trophoblast invasion to flourish. A number of researchers and clinicians now believe that some cases of recurrent miscarriage are due to the mother's immune system releasing raised levels of NK cells that attack the fetus, possibly because of genetic mutations in the HLA gene and a failure to produce 'blocking factors' to protect the fetus. However, there is no direct scientific evidence to support this theory, and successful pregnancies can occur in the absence of 'blocking' antibody.[15] Furthermore, there is little evidence that uNK cells attack placental or embryonic cells.

In the first trimester, placental tissues are very sensitive to oxidative stress, due to a low concentration of antioxidants. Recent research in the UK[15] suggests that the increased density of uNK cells noted in many studies of RM and implantation failure may contribute to the promotion of angiogenesis, and consequently endometrial blood flow, leading to excessive oxidative stress in the early placenta, and subsequent miscarriage. This would be consistent with data from other researchers which demonstrates higher than normal placental oxidative stress, trophoblast degeneration and disrupted circulation in miscarried pregnancies.[16] Findings from other studies point to a spectrum of disorder for pregnancies that do continue. Defects in placentation are known to be involved in pre-eclampsia, many cases of intrauterine growth restriction (IUGR), premature labour and stillbirth.[17]

Despite the many studies that have examined the role of the immune system in pregnancy loss, research findings are contradictory and there is still no clear pathological model. At the present time experts only seem to agree universally on one thing, namely that immune dysfunction in one form or another is at least partly responsible for some cases of pregnancy loss.

Autoimmune factors
Antiphospholipid syndrome
In autoimmune reactions, the body attacks itself through the production of antibodies. Over the past few years, this has emerged as one of the few unequivocal treatable mechanisms underlying some cases of RM. Two of the most common antiphospholipids (aPL) are lupus anticoagulant and anticardiolipin antibody, and both are involved in RM. Antiphospholipid syndrome (APS) causes miscarriage through several mechanisms, and is known to cause different problems at different gestational stages. It was

initially thought that it was only responsible for late miscarriages as a result of the thrombophilic changes in the uteroplacental vessels. 'Sticky blood' forms clots in the placenta, which if the pregnancy survived would also be associated with pre-eclampsia, premature labour and IUGR. Nowadays it is known that APS is directly responsible for non-thrombotic attacks on the development of the placenta, including hostile inflammatory reactions and inhibition of the release of hCG by placental cells, and causes pregnancy loss from the earliest gestational stage, namely implantation.

Thyroid antibodies

It is possible to have thyroid antibodies even with a normally functioning thyroid, and a finding of raised antibodies alone is not an indication that the woman will go on to develop thyroid problems or pregnancy complications. However, recurrent miscarriage sufferers do have a higher prevalence of thyroid antibodies, and some clinicians may decide to investigate further, although as yet a definitive association between this and an increased incidence of miscarriage remains unconfirmed.

THROMBOPHILIAS

Thrombophilias that are implicated in pregnancy loss, particularly RM, can be classified as hereditary and acquired, principally antiphospholipid syndrome.

Hereditary thrombophilias

Hereditary thrombophilias are a group of genetic coagulation disorders. Specific gene mutations make the carriers more susceptible to developing thrombosis, and although not everyone with a blood-clotting disorder will experience pregnancy loss or any clinical manifestations at all, a number of studies demonstrate strong associations with obstetric complications, including late miscarriage (see Box 2.1). Thrombophilias increase the risk of placental abruption, IUGR, severe pre-eclampsia, iatrogenic preterm labour, excessive intrapartum and postpartum haemorrhage, antenatal and postpartum deep vein thrombophlebitis and pulmonary embolism.[3] Although there are known links between hereditary clotting disorders and pregnancy loss, this alone does not determine which women will develop pregnancy complications. It is apparent from the data currently available that multiple factors are involved in determining who is affected. Identification of a specific gene mutation in an individual may not necessarily provide the single reason (or treatment) for their pregnancy loss.

BOX 2.1: Hereditary thrombophilias associated with obstetric complications

Antithrombin III deficiency Prevalence of around 1 in 600 of the population; carries a 50% lifetime risk of thrombosis; associated with miscarriage and stillbirth

Protein C deficiency Prevalence of around 1 in 500 of the population; levels remain unaltered in pregnancy

Protein S deficiency Around 0.03–0.13% of the population is affected; acts as a cofactor for the action of protein C; levels fall in pregnancy

Factor V Leiden mutation Around 5% of Caucasians are affected; prevalence is highest in Europeans (rarely found in other racial groups); increased incidence of late pregnancy complications, including severe pre-eclampsia, placental abruption, fetal loss and lower live birth rates

Prothrombin gene mutation Present in around 2–3% of the population; an association has been shown with placental disruption and second-trimester losses

Hyperhomocysteinaemia Associated with folate deficiency, neural tube defects, pre-eclampsia, placental abruption, fetal growth restriction and recurrent miscarriage

---

INFECTIOUS CAUSES

Infections are associated with adverse pregnancy outcomes, including early or late miscarriages, stillbirths, neonatal and childhood problems (*see* Box 2.2). Although minor infections are unlikely to cause serious complications, physiological maternal immunosuppression that occurs in pregnancy can lead to higher rates of bacterial and viral infections and associated problems. Bacterial vaginosis affects around 20% of pregnant women and is associated with preterm delivery, second-trimester miscarriage, amniotic fluid infection and chorioamnionitis.[10]

For an infectious cause to be implicated in RM, the infection must persist and be present in each pregnancy. However, such infections are rare. At one time, TORCH screening was routinely advised for women who experienced more than one miscarriage, but this approach has now been abandoned in mainstream medical investigations. TORCH is an acronym for the following group of infections:

➤ Toxoplasmosis
➤ Other infections (e.g. congenital syphilis, viral infections)
➤ Rubella
➤ Cytomegalovirus
➤ Herpes simplex virus.

BOX 2.2: Infections and organisms associated with pregnancy loss and obstetric and neonatal complications

Bacterial infections
• Group B streptococcus
• Chorioamnionitis
• *Listeria* species
• Bacterial vaginosis
• Gonorrhoea
• Chlamydia
• Tuberculosis

Protozoal infections
• Toxoplasmosis
• Trichomoniasis

Viral infections
• Rubella
• Cytomegalovirus

Spirochaetes
• Syphilis
• Lyme disease

ENVIRONMENTAL CAUSES

There are abundant alarmist stories about the perils of our modern world and lifestyles and their impact on our health. As a practitioner of natural medicine I have firmly retained a degree of criticality in reviewing the literature on possible environmental causes of miscarriage. In complementary medicine there is often an inherent bias towards promoting health through methods that are more in tune with natural philosophy, rather than at odds with the environment. This makes it easy to adopt the default position of assuming that environmental factors must be to blame for health concerns, including miscarriage. However, much of the evidence for associations between specific environmental factors and pregnancy loss is contradictory, although many of these factors remain of concern. Although numerous factors have been implicated in miscarriage studies, there are several problems with many of these reports that make it difficult to draw firm conclusions about cause rather than association. A major problem is that once a specific factor is suspected, control groups are often difficult to establish. Of the several hundred suspected environmental factors, only a very few have been identified through robust studies as being damaging to pregnancy.

Reports of apparent 'clusters' of miscarriage linked either geographically or by some other association, such as occupation, can readily be found in the literature, especially in the less scientifically rigorous works. The often alarmist nature of reporting on environmental links to miscarriage ensures that whatever 'culprit' is under discussion is long afterwards perceived to be guilty even if it is later disproven. For many of the reports and studies that have been published over the years and that have entered the popular mind, closer scrutiny typically reveals flaws in study design, confounding variables, or studies producing different conclusions. However, these criticisms and alternative perspectives rarely receive much attention, and in the minds of women (and some professionals) the 'villains' continue to be held responsible for pregnancy losses. A thorough and convincing examination of the problems can be found in the discussion in Jon Cohen's *Coming to Term*.[4]

Cigarettes and alcohol

The examples of alcohol and smoking illustrate some of the difficulties with studies in the field. Although it is known that a heavy and regular alcohol intake increases the risks of both early and late miscarriages, due to its teratogenic and toxic effects on the developing baby, studies can be problematic, as heavy drinkers are often also smokers, and it is difficult to separate the effects of each of these factors. One of the largest studies on smoking that adjusted for alcohol use found an increase in miscarriage rates only among women who smoked heavily. Mothers who smoke during pregnancy have a significantly increased risk of preterm delivery and fetal growth restriction. A large study of Swedish women reported that women who stopped smoking reduced their risk of stillbirth, thus providing strong evidence that maternal smoking during pregnancy is causally associated with stillbirth risk.[18]

According to a recent UK report on stillbirth and infant mortality trends, a high proportion of mothers under the age of 20 years are smokers, with the highest rates seen among European and Afro-Caribbean ethnic groups, and the lowest rates found in Asian women.[19] It is known that smoking reduces the delivery of oxygen and nutrients to the baby as well as having adverse effects on female and male reproductive health generally. This is a preventable cause of stillbirth, preterm delivery and miscarriage, and so without doubt couples must be counselled to stop smoking before conception if they wish to minimise the risks to the baby.

The safety of alcohol in pregnancy is more complicated in some respects, and women are often confused by conflicting reports of apparently safe levels of alcohol that appear in the media from time to time. Maternal nutrition is adversely affected if the woman consumes alcohol, as the latter interferes with the absorption of some nutrients. Although the teratogenic effect of alcohol is dose-related, the exact level at which alcohol causes harm varies with each individual. Therefore it is sensible to advise women that no safe level of alcohol consumption in pregnancy has been established, and that alcohol is thus best avoided. However, for the concerned woman who had a few drinks before she discovered that she was pregnant, reassurance should be given that the risk to the baby is extremely low, and a strenuous effort should be made to reduce any anxiety arising from this.

> Kate, who had been trying to conceive for two years following a late miscarriage, came to me racked with guilt and fear on discovering the happy news that she was pregnant, following a weekend away celebrating her fortieth birthday, at which she had allowed herself for the first time in two years to have a few drinks during the course of the weekend. Subsequently she discovered that she was pregnant, but instead of feeling optimism and joy, she was plagued by weeks of guilt and fear. She went on to deliver a healthy

girl with no pregnancy complications, but only at around 28 weeks did she forgive herself for drinking that champagne.

Substance abuse

Recreational drugs are not good for any person, including pregnant women and their unborn children, and should not be used, irrespective of the proven or unproven obstetric hazards. Abusing any substance undoubtedly increases the risk of pregnancy complications and damage to the developing baby. Different substances will cause damage in different ways, but some of the more commonly used substances and their known obstetric effects include the following.

Cocaine

Cocaine decreases uterine blood flow and increases uterine vascular resistance, and has possible teratogenic effects, leading to congenital malformations. As it is metabolised by plasma and liver cholinesterase, the levels of which drop during pregnancy, it has increased toxicity during pregnancy for both mother and fetus. It also stimulates uterine contractions, and there is a higher incidence of placental abruption and stillbirth in users.

Heroin

Heroin-specific problems are difficult to assess, as users frequently abuse more than one substance and have multiple health and socio-economic problems. The most common reproductive disorder is infertility, as heroin is known to inhibit ovulation. Maternal heroin use has been associated with increased risks of preterm labour, pre-eclampsia, postpartum haemorrhage and IUGR.

Marijuana

Reports suggest that this is the most commonly used recreational drug among women of childbearing age,[3] and it is known to inhibit ovulation and adversely affect male fertility. Little is known about its teratogenic effects.

Caffeine

Caffeine has long been implicated in miscarriage, but until recently studies have produced conflicting results. The latest research has confirmed that too much caffeine can not only result in an increased likelihood of miscarriage, but may also lead to lower birth weights.[20,21] The UK's Food Standards Agency revised its recommendations in 2008 to advise pregnant women to limit their daily caffeine intake, ideally to below 200 mg a day. Caffeine is found not only in coffee and tea, but also in chocolate and some soft drinks.

Nutrition
Body mass index (BMI)
Both under- and overweight women are at higher risk of miscarriage than those of normal weight, and maternal pre-conception body mass index (BMI) has been shown to be a risk factor for stillbirths for women with a BMI of less than 18.5 or greater than 25 kg/m².[22] Low BMI may be an indicator for low vitamin intake and poor diet generally, which may account for it being an apparent risk factor for first-trimester miscarriage.[23] Furthermore, some research suggests that the increased risk of miscarriage may be associated with impaired endometrial function rather than with poor embryo quality, as studies of egg donation IVF cycles, where only good-quality embryos are used, show a correlation with BMI and miscarriage rates.[24]

Diet
Much has been written about nutrition and pregnancy, and a whole industry supports the view that a balanced diet alone is insufficient in our modern world, and that vitamin supplementation is necessary to maximise health. However, although poor diet with insufficient nutritional value is associated with pregnancy loss, supplementing with vitamins has not been shown to reduce the number of women who miscarry or have a stillbirth.[25] This finding is interesting, as it supports the view held in traditional Chinese medicine (TCM) that good health depends upon a diet that supports our digestive system, which in turn is central to our well-being, and no amount of supplementation alone will compensate for a poor diet.

A recent UK population-based study that examined risk factors for first-trimester miscarriages identified that eating fresh fruit and vegetables daily had an apparently protective effect for women.[23] Although a good balanced diet will sustain a healthy pregnancy, the following foods must be avoided, as they may cause serious complications in pregnancy:
➤ uncooked or soft cooked eggs, or products containing these
➤ unpasteurised milk and soft cheeses made with this

➤ undercooked meat, poultry and shellfish
➤ meat and vegetarian pâtés
➤ liver and liver products.

Folic acid supplementation has been standard medical advice for some time for pregnant women and those trying to conceive, as low levels of folic acid are implicated in the development of neural tube defects (NTD) in children. Women should increase their daily intake of folic acid by 0.4 mg before pregnancy and throughout the first trimester. There is an additional reason why this is good advice, that is specifically associated with miscarriage. Inherited hyperhomocysteinaemia, an inherited thrombophilia, results in folate deficiency and is associated with RM as well as with NTD. Although the mechanisms involved are unclear, it is thought that the condition leads to impaired development of placental blood vessels. Therefore, although it is still the subject of some debate, the recommendation to ensure adequate folate intake may have benefits beyond the prevention of NTD. Furthermore, recent research has identified a significant association with male folate intake and sperm aneuploidy. Although the design of this particular study did not allow causality to be established, the findings warrant further research.[26]

Radiation and X-rays

Exposure to high doses of radiation definitely harms the fetus and has long-term effects on parental health, including fertility. However, having an occasional X-ray presents an extremely low risk to any developing fetus, so undue concern should not arise unless a long series of X-rays were undertaken in the first trimester, and even then the risk to the pregnancy is small. Cosmic radiation exposure, as occurs during high-altitude flying, has been studied as a concern not only for travellers, but also for those working in the airline industry. Current data suggest that, for pregnant women, the risk posed to casual air travellers of direct harm from cosmic radiation is negligible, and even for those with more frequent exposure, such as aircrew and frequent business travellers, the risks appear to be inconsequential.[27]

OTHER RISK FACTORS
Maternal age
Both of the extreme ends of the age range are associated with preterm delivery and low birth weight, and older mothers have a higher incidence of antenatal complications such as essential hypertension, pre-eclampsia, gestational diabetes and placental abruption, all of which are known to contribute to stillbirth.[22] Advanced maternal age has also been reported as a risk factor for stillbirth and neonatal death. This is independent of confounding factors such as hypertension, diabetes and assisted conception, with mothers over 35 years of age having an increased risk, which rises for those aged over 40 years.[28,29] Maternal age below 20 years is associated with an increased incidence of neonatal death, which may be linked to socio-economic factors such as higher rates of deprivation in this age group and an increased risk of preterm delivery.[22] Research published in 2005[30] found an increased risk of spontaneous miscarriage in the first trimester among women aged below 20 or over 35 years, confirming the findings of several previous studies that demonstrated a higher risk in teenage pregnancies.

Occupational hazards
It has long been recognised that the working habits and environment of a pregnant woman might affect her pregnancy outcome, and statutory rights to maternity leave and other concessions in the workplace are testament to this recognition. The precise extent to which working patterns and types of work affect pregnancy, and the mechanisms involved, are not fully understood, and as with many of the suspected causes of adverse pregnancy outcomes, studies in this area are difficult to undertake, as variables are difficult to control for and most of the published data come from observational studies. However, numerous adequately designed studies[31-33] have shown associations between preterm birth, low birth weight and miscarriage for the following working conditions:
- shift work and night work
- demanding working postures for at least 3 hours per day
- work that results in whole-body vibrations
- psychosocial stress at work
- physically demanding work and prolonged standing
- high cumulative work fatigue.

Possible mechanisms that have been proposed through which adverse pregnancy outcomes may occur include effects mediated by the sympathetic nervous system, with the release of prostaglandins and stress hormones such as catecholamines into the maternal circulation, which may lead to increases in blood pressure, uterine contractility and decreased placental function.[33] It is also worth considering that although these conditions have been studied within the field of employment, some of these factors may occur in regular domestic life for some women, especially those with lower socio-economic status, for whom demanding domestic work may be routine.

There are many jobs that involve exposure to potentially harmful chemicals, and pregnancy and reproductive outcomes have been studied in groups of workers in a variety of industries and professions, including hairdressing, dental work, various industrial manufacturing processes, pharmacies, laboratories and farming, among many others. There is no doubt that exposure to certain chemicals prior to or during pregnancy may have serious consequences. However, modern industrial practices and legislation that protect the health of workers are in place to minimise, if not entirely eliminate, the risks posed to them. Women should be encouraged to be aware of protective practices within their workplace, to enable preventive action to be initiated with regard to any threat posed to their pregnancy by their working environment.

Maternal stress and psychological factors

It has long been postulated that maternal psychological stress may affect pregnancy outcome, and recent studies have confirmed this long-held belief.[34-36] Several papers have highlighted associations between preterm labour and stressful life events, anxiety, depression, stressful work, being in physically abusive relationships and having low levels of social support.[37] It has been suggested that depression prior to conception is correlated with higher rates of miscarriage in women experiencing RM. The relatively new scientific field of psychoneuroimmunology (PNI) has shown that complex communication pathways operate between the psycho-neuro-immuno-endocrine interfaces, and may in time lead to a fuller understanding of the causal pathways of adverse pregnancy outcome.[35]

Multiple pregnancies

Compared with single pregnancies, multiple pregnancies have a higher risk of complications during pregnancy and after birth. Problems with growth, preterm delivery and higher levels of stillbirth and neonatal deaths in twins and higher-order multiples have been reported.[22] With the advent of assisted conception, there has been a concurrent increase in multiple pregnancy rates in developed countries. These topics are covered in detail in Chapter 3.

OTHER SUSPECTED CAUSES

I am regularly asked by my patients about my views on a range of things that they have read or heard are likely to be harmful to their pregnancies, and I always advise them that if something is not good for their general health, it is to be avoided as far as is practical. In addition, there are a few specific things to cut out. These are based upon my understanding of where the evidence is most persuasive and the experts largely agree, as well as my experience as a natural health practitioner. My perspective, like that of many involved in complementary medicine, is always that the less exposure we have to artificial, synthesised chemicals, the healthier we and the planet will be, but I am also a pragmatist, and I try to encourage my patients to adopt a balanced perspective on what to do, eat, drink or use and what is best avoided. Some of the most commonly discussed concerns among my patients, and those often cited on the Internet and in less critically evaluated literature, are listed in Box 2.3.

BOX 2.3: Frequently cited or suspected causes of pregnancy loss which lack supporting evidence

- Air travel
- Exercise
- Hair colourants
- Hot tubs
- Massage
- Microwave ovens
- Mobile phones
- Saunas
- Ultrasound scans
- Video display units (VDUs)

In the case of most of these frequently cited or suspected causes, large research studies have been conducted which have disproved any link between their use and pregnancy loss. Others remain scientifically unexplored, often due to lack of research funding or interest. However, anxieties persist well beyond the initial scare stories which bring them to public attention in the first place. For example, consider air travel. I am very often asked about this, and I always suggest that patients check with their doctors, but I am certain from reading the literature that it poses no more risk (in fact probably less) than travelling on a train. However, many advise against it during the first trimester, despite the fact that there is no evidence at all that it disturbs an otherwise healthy pregnancy.[38] In fact, an interesting finding from an exploratory study of risk factors for first-trimester losses found a striking reduction in the incidence of miscarriage in women who flew during the first 12 weeks of pregnancy compared with those who avoided flying.[23] However, it would seem prudent to avoid flying during pregnancy if there are concurrent medical conditions that may be worsened by the hypoxic environment of an aeroplane, such as cardiopulmonary disorders, or if a woman is known to be at risk of preterm labour or has any identified placental pathology or history of thrombosis.

STILLBIRTH AND INTRAUTERINE DEATH

The causes of stillbirth are varied and often difficult to determine, with no obvious reason for a late fetal death. Many stillbirths are completely unexpected and occur in women who are in good health and who have had otherwise normal pregnancies. According to the International Stillbirth Alliance, 4.5 million stillbirths occur each year around the world, with the rate in developed countries estimated to be one in 100–200 pregnancies.[39] The most recent data from the UK's Confidential Enquiry into Maternal and Child Health show that almost 75% of stillbirths in 2007 were unexplained[22] (*see* Box 2.4).

BOX 2.4: Cause-of-death classification of stillbirths in the UK in 2007[22]

- Congenital anomaly (0.1%)
- Pre-eclampsia (4.9%)
- Antepartum haemorrhage (10.7%)

- Mechanical causes (1.5%)
- Maternal disorder (8.1%)
- Miscellaneous (0.2%)
- Unexplained (74.4%)

Post-mortem examinations can potentially help to increase understanding of the causes of stillbirth, but in 2007 only 45% of stillbirths underwent post-mortem examination. Only in exceptional circumstances (e.g. a coroner's investigation) are post-mortems carried out without parental consent, which is required under UK law for all live births and those legally classified as stillborn (i.e. after 24 weeks' gestation). Although some parents will regard a post-mortem as an opportunity to find out why their baby died and whether there are implications for future pregnancies, others will be unable to move beyond their shock and distress and will refuse to give their consent, or will object to a post-mortem on grounds of religion or culture. The relatively low post-mortem rate has been attributed to the difficulty of discussing this issue with bereaved parents in the emotional aftermath of the birth. This is not helped by uninformed or inexpert staff being allocated the difficult task of obtaining consent. Furthermore, the personal or religious objections of parents may hinder the process.[40]

REFERENCES

1 Wilson R. *Recurrent Miscarriage and Pre-Eclampsia.* London: Imperial College Press; 2004.

2 Farquharson RG, ed. *Miscarriage.* Dinton, Wiltshire: Mark Allen Publishing; 2002.

3 Gilbert E, Harmon J. *Manual of High Risk Pregnancy and Delivery.* 3rd edn. St Louis, MO: Mosby; 2003.

4 Cohen J. *Coming to Term.* New Brunswick, NJ: Rutgers University Press; 2007.

5 de la Rochebrochard E, Thonneau P. Paternal age and maternal age are risk factors for miscarriage: results of a multicentre European study. *Human Reproduction* 2002; **17**: 1649–56.

6 Kleinhaus K, Perrin M, Friedlander Y *et al.* Paternal age and spontaneous abortion. *Obstetrics and Gynecology* 2006; **108**: 369–77.

7 Kushnir VA, Scott RT, Frattarelli JL. Effect of paternal age on aneuploidy rates in first trimester pregnancy loss. *Journal of Medical Genetics and Genomics* 2010; **2**: 38–43.

8   Regan L. *Miscarriage: what every woman needs to know.* London: Orion; 2001.

9   Danielsson K. *After Miscarriage: medical facts and emotional support for pregnancy loss.* Boston, MA: Harvard Common Press; 2008.

10 James DK, Steer PJ, Weiner CP *et al. High Risk Pregnancy Management Options.* 3rd edn. Philadelphia, PA: Elsevier; 2006.

11 Saravelos SH, Cocksedge KA, Li TC. Prevalence and diagnosis of congenital uterine anomalies in women with reproductive failure: a critical appraisal. *Human Reproduction Update* 2008; **14:** 415–29.

12 Edmonds DK. *Dewhurst's Textbook of Obstetrics and Gynaecology.* 7th edn. Oxford: Blackwell Publishing; 2007.

13 National Institute for Health and Clinical Excellence (NICE). *IPG228. Laparoscopic Cerclage for Prevention of Recurrent Pregnancy Loss due to Cervical Incompetence: guidance.* London: NICE; 2007. http://guidance.nice.org.uk/IPG228/Guidance/pdf/English

14 Glueck CJ, Wang P, Goldenberg N *et al.* Pregnancy outcomes among women with polycystic ovary syndrome treated with metformin. *Human Reproduction* 2002; **17:** 2858–64.

15 Royal College of Obstetricians and Gynaecologists. *Immunological Testing and Interventions for Reproductive Failure.* Scientific Advisory Committee Opinion Paper 5. London: Royal College of Obstetricians and Gynaecologists; 2008.

16 Quenby S, Nik H, Innes B *et al.* Early pregnancy uterine natural killer cells and angiogenesis in recurrent reproductive failure. *Human Reproduction* 2009; **24:** 45–54.

17 Hiby SE, Regan L, Lo W *et al.* Association of maternal killer-cell immunoglobulin-like receptors and parental HLA-C genotypes with recurrent miscarriage. *Human Reproduction* 2008; **23:** 972–6.

18 Högberg L, Cnattingius S. The influence of maternal smoking habits on the risk of subsequent stillbirth: is there a causal relation? *British Journal of Obstetrics and Gynaecology* 2007; **114:** 699–704.

19 Gardosi J, Beamish N, Francis A *et al. Stillbirth and Infant Mortality, West Midlands 1997–2005: trends, factors, inequalities.* Birmingham: West Midlands Perinatal Institute; 2007. www.perinatal.nhs.uk/pnm/WM_SB&IMR_2007report.pdf (accessed 30 November 2009).

20 Weng X, Odouli R, Li DK. Maternal caffeine consumption during pregnancy and the risk of miscarriage: a prospective cohort study. *American Journal of Obstetrics and Gynecology* 2008; **198:** 279. e1–8.

21 CARE Study Group. Maternal caffeine intake during pregnancy and risk of fetal growth restriction: a large prospective observational study. *BMJ* 2008; **337:** a2332.

22 Confidential Enquiry into Maternal and Child Health (CEMACH). *Perinatal Mortality 2007: United Kingdom.* London: CEMACH; 2009.

23 Maconochie N, Doyle P, Prior S *et al*. Risk factors for first trimester miscarriage – results from a UK-population-based case–control study. *British Journal of Obstetrics and Gynaecology* 2007; **114**: 170–86.

24 Veleva Z, Tiitinen A, Vilska S *et al*. High and low BMI increase the risk of miscarriage after IVF/ICSI and FET. *Human Reproduction* 2008; **23**: 878–84.

25 Rumbold A, Middleton P, Crowther CA. Vitamin supplementation for preventing miscarriage. *Cochrane Database of Systematic Reviews* 2005; **2**: CD004073.

26 Young SS, Eskenazi B, Marchetti FM *et al*. The association of folate, zinc and antioxidant intake with sperm aneuploidy in healthy non-smoking men. *Human Reproduction* 2008; **23**: 1014–22.

27 Barish RJ. In-flight radiation exposure during pregnancy. *Obstetrics and Gynecology* 2004; **103**: 1326–30.

28 Hoffman MC, Jeffers S, Carter J *et al*. Pregnancy at or beyond age 40 years is associated with an increased risk of fetal death and other adverse outcomes. *American Journal of Obstetrics and Gynecology* 2007; **196**: e11–13.

29 Delbaerea I, Verstraelena H, Goetgelukb S *et al*. Pregnancy outcome in primiparae of advanced maternal age. *European Journal of Obstetrics, Gynecology and Reproductive Biology* 2007; **135**: 41–6.

30 Gracia CR, Sammel MD, Chittams J *et al*. Risk factors for spontaneous abortion in early symptomatic first-trimester pregnancies. *Obstetrics and Gynecology* 2005; **106**: 993–9.

31 Croteau A, Marcoux S, Brisson C. Work activity in pregnancy, preventive measures and the risk of preterm delivery. *American Journal of Epidemiology* 2007; **166**: 951–65.

32 Knutsson A. Health disorders of shift workers. *Occupational Medicine* 2003; **53**: 103–8.

33 Mozurkewich EL, Luke B, Avni M *et al*. Working conditions and adverse pregnancy outcome: a meta-analysis. *Obstetrics and Gynecology* 2000; **95**: 623–35.

34 Field T, Diego M, Hernandez-Reif M. Prenatal depression effects on the fetus and newborn: a review. *Infant Behavior and Development* 2006; **29**: 445–55.

35 Van den Bergh BRH, Mulder EJH, Mennes M *et al*. Antenatal maternal anxiety and stress and the neurobehavioural development of the fetus and child: links and possible mechanisms. A review. *Neuroscience and Biobehavioral Reviews* 2005; **29**: 237–58.

36 Mulder EJH, Robles de Medina PG, Huizink AC *et al*. Prenatal maternal stress: effects on pregnancy and the (unborn) child. *Early Human Development* 2002; **70**: 3–14.

37 Kramer MS, Goulet L, Lydon J. Socio-economic disparities in preterm birth: causal pathways and mechanisms. *Paediatric and Perinatal Epidemiology* 2001; **15 (Suppl. 2)**: 104–23.

38 Koren G. Is air travel in pregnancy safe? *Canadian Family Physician* 2008; **54**: 1241–2.

39 www.stillbirthalliance.org

40 Royal College of Obstetricians and Gynaecologists. *Fetal and Perinatal Pathology. Report of a Joint Working Party.* London: RCOG Press; 2001.

CHAPTER 3

Multiple pregnancy and infertility

INTRODUCTION

In general, during pregnancy a woman's body undergoes a physiologically normal, albeit quite remarkable event. However, there are a number of factors that can complicate pregnancies, leading to a minority of women being identified as 'high risk', where the likelihood of an adverse outcome to the pregnancy is greater than that for the general population. With the dramatic increase in the incidence of multiple births in the past few decades, which is concordant with the wider use of fertility treatments, this chapter gives these topics special attention. Nearly every obstetric complication occurs more frequently in multiple pregnancies, and perinatal mortality is nearly four times higher in twins and six times higher in triplets than in singletons.[1] However, it must be emphasised that the risks associated with multiple pregnancies rarely arise from the infertility treatments. Almost all of the complications of multiple pregnancy occur in both spontaneous and assisted conceptions.[2]

Whether or not the incidence of miscarriage and pregnancy loss is higher in those undergoing assisted reproductive treatment (ART) is a question that many studies have investigated, but which remains open.[3] Although there is some evidence which suggests that the risk of miscarriage is higher than in natural conceptions, the comparison is problematic, as ART pregnancies tend to be under immediate scrutiny, so losses can be detected and reported at a very early stage. Furthermore, as a selected group, women undergoing ART may have features that predispose them to an increased risk of miscarriage. Of these, advanced age is the most likely characteristic that has been identified as influencing pregnancy outcome.

MULTIPLE PREGNANCY
Aetiology
The most common multiple is a twin pregnancy, with higher-order multiples (three or more fetuses) being much rarer. The majority of twins (75%) are dizygotic (DZ) and result from the fertilisation of two ova by two sperm. Monozygotic (MZ) twins (i.e. identical twins) arise from the splitting of a single fertilised ovum. The natural occurrence of DZ twins has a hereditary component, and the incidence is higher among women in certain ethnic groups, with increasing parity and maternal age, whereas the incidence of MZ remains constant around the world at 4 per 1000 births. The greatest risk of complication in multiple pregnancy is determined by chorionicity rather than zygosity.[4]

Chorionicity and zygosity
All DZ pregnancies are dichorionic (DC) with two separate placentas. This presents lesser risk than that experienced by the majority of MZ twins. In MZ pregnancies, the fetal membranes may surround one or more of the fetuses and they can have shared or separate placentas. Chorionicity relates to the placentation of the pregnancy, and is determined by the stage at which the zygote divides (*see* Figure 3.1). The later this occurs in embryonic development, the greater the potential for problems, as more structures are shared. Around a third of MZ twins establish before the third day after fertilisation,

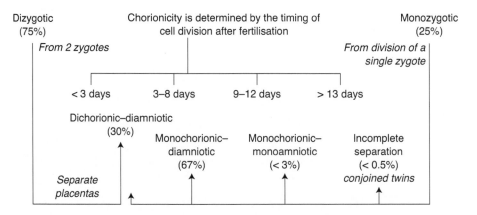

FIGURE 3.1: Zygosity and chorionicity in twin pregnancies with relative frequencies.

so that two separate blastocysts form and implant with a separate placenta and amniotic sac for each twin. This is known as *dichorionic diamniotic placentation*. Most of the remaining MZ twins develop after the third day, resulting in *monochorionic diamniotic placentation*, where a single placenta supports two fetuses but they have separate amniotic sacs. Much more rarely, later cleavage after day nine produces a single amniotic cavity, resulting in *monochorionic monoamniotic* twins. Monochorionic placentation can also occur in higher-order multiples.

Complications of multiple pregnancy

All the normal maternal physiological adaptations of pregnancy increase in multiple pregnancies, as do the risks of any pregnancy complication, such as hypertension, placental abruption and anaemia. In addition, there are certain problems that are specific to multiple pregnancies that can threaten the outcome (*see* Table 3.1). Preterm delivery is the greatest risk, and its incidence rises as fetal number increases. Many of the health problems associated with twins are due to their higher risk of being born prematurely.

TABLE 3.1: Risks and complications in multiple pregnancies

Maternal problems	Fetal problems
Anaemia	Congenital anomalies
Gestational diabetes	Discordant growth*
Hyperemesis gravidarum	Growth restriction
Placenta abruption	Intrauterine fetal death
Placenta previa	Twin–twin transfusion syndrome*
Postpartum haemorrhage	'Vanishing twin' phenomenon*
Pre-eclampsia	Umbilical cord entanglement
Pregnancy-induced hypertension	
Premature rupture of membranes	
Preterm labour	
Spontaneous early miscarriage	

* Only occur in multiple pregnancy.

Fetal complications

Multiplets have a more complicated life *in utero* than singletons and, as previously mentioned, monozygotic twins are at higher risk than dizygotic twins, but it is chorionicity and amnionicity rather than zygosity that determines the degree of risk. The particular challenges of a monochorionic (MC) pregnancy arise from the unique structure of the shared placenta, with vascular structures connecting the umbilical circulations of both twins. This leads to unpredictable and significant blood volume shifts between the fetuses causing problems such as twin–twin transfusion and acute fetal transfusion following the intrauterine death of one twin. Furthermore, the shared placenta is often unequally divided, which explains the increased incidence of discordant fetal growth. Perinatal mortality is two to three times higher in MC twins than in DC twins, and morbidity rates are similarly raised.[1]

Intrauterine fetal death

Perinatal mortality statistics do not accurately reflect the problems of multiple pregnancies, because the highest rate of fetal loss occurs prior to viability. Monochorionic twins have a six times higher fetal loss rate (12%) between 10 and 24 weeks' gestation compared with dichorionic twins and singletons.[4] Furthermore, it is estimated that around 20% of twin pregnancies end in the early resorption of one fetus previously seen on ultrasound, which is known as the 'vanishing twin' phenomenon. However, this may not provide a truly accurate picture of the degree of pregnancy loss that multiples present, as the death of one fetus, a single intrauterine death (sIUFD), may occur before the diagnosis of multiple pregnancy has been made and may therefore go unrecognised.

The prognosis with regard to sIUFD for the remaining fetus is strongly dependent on chorionicity and amnionicity. The intrauterine death of both fetuses is more common than sIUFD in monochorionic twins, due to the shared fetoplacental circulation. Haemodynamic imbalances, chromosomal abnormalities and adverse maternal factors such as infection will tend to affect both twins. In contrast, the separate circulations that are characteristic of dichorionic twins means that sIUFD does not necessarily lead to double IUFD, and the outcome is often positive, although if the sIUFD occurs towards the end of the first trimester, rates of miscarriage and preterm delivery of the remaining twin are increased.

Chorionicity can be identified by ultrasound assessment of the dividing membranes before 14 weeks' gestation with almost 100% accuracy in the first trimester. Correct determination of chorionicity is important, as increased monitoring may improve the outcome. In the past, maternal management was the priority, but with advances in ultrasound technology the modern approach emphasises recognising the fetal risk as determined by chorionicity, monitoring fetal growth and well-being by ultrasound scanning, and reducing the risks of preterm delivery.[1]

Maternal complications

All maternal organ systems are required to adapt to the demands of pregnancy, and these normal physiological adaptations in the mother are heightened in multiple pregnancy:

➤ Renal blood flow increases.
➤ Systemic vascular resistance decreases.
➤ Cardiac output increases.
➤ Red cell mass increases by around 300 ml more than in singletons, but haemoglobin values fall.

As well as the increased demands arising from these normal maternal responses, gestational diabetes, hyperemesis gravidarum and pre-eclampsia are all more common in multiple pregnancies, and in the case of the latter two can be more severe. Larger uterine size contributes to an increase in the severity of other common pregnancy-related problems, such as varicose veins, backache, oedema, haemorrhoids and heartburn, and the physical discomfort reported by women is often considerable towards the end of the pregnancy.

Preterm labour

Preterm labour (PTL) can be defined as regular uterine contractions that cause progressive dilation of the cervix after 24 weeks' gestation and before 37 weeks. The risk increases as fetal number increases (*see* Figure 3.2), and prematurity is the leading cause of neonatal death in multiple pregnancy, accounting for 85% of all perinatal morbidity and mortality.[5] As well as multiple pregnancy, a number of other risk factors for preterm labour have been identified (*see* Box 3.1), but in over 50% of cases the causes remain unknown.[5,6]

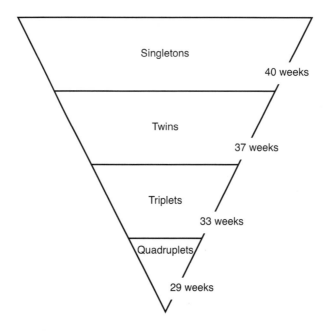

FIGURE 3.2: Average length of gestation in multiple pregnancy.

BOX 3.1: Risk factors for preterm labour

Obstetric and gynaecological factors
- Cervical or uterine anomalies
- Intra-amniotic infection
- Multiple pregnancy
- Placental abruption
- Polyhydramnios
- Premature rupture of membranes
- Prior preterm birth
- Second- or third-trimester bleeding
- Vaginal infections, especially bacterial vaginosis

Medical factors
- Anaemia
- Cardiovascular disease
- Diabetes
- Hypertension

- Renal disease
- Urinary tract infection

Environmental, social and demographic factors
- Afro-Caribbean ethnicity
- BMI $< 19\,\text{kg/m}^2$
- Domestic violence
- Extreme maternal age (under 20 or over 35 years)
- High levels of physical and/or emotional stress
- Low socio-economic status
- Physically demanding work involving prolonged standing and shift work
- Smoking and alcohol abuse
- Use of recreational drugs (especially cocaine)

Preventing preterm labour

In multiple pregnancy, PTL is increased by over-distension of the uterus and, strictly speaking, there are no specific preventive measures that can modify this risk apart from fetal reduction in higher-order multiples. Despite the lack of evidence supporting its use, hospitalised bed rest has been a regular practice for many years. It is useful for practitioners to do what they can to lower the risk to each woman as far as possible by adopting a holistic approach to her care. In addition to raising the woman's awareness of the signs and symptoms of PTL, relevant healthcare practitioners can actively assist by assessing and intervening appropriately if additional risk factors are identified (*see* Box 3.1).

Instructing the mother to be alert for the signs and symptoms of PTL is worthwhile, but it can be difficult to identify in multiple pregnancy, as these signs and symptoms can easily be mistaken for the extra aches, pains and pressure with which the woman is probably already familiar. However, if she is made as aware as possible of the symptoms and signs of PTL, the woman can be advised to present early if it is suspected. It is important that she feels comfortable about reporting any signs of PTL and is encouraged to do so with open communication. Symptoms that should be reported include:
➤ menstrual-like cramps
➤ dull lower backache
➤ pelvic pressure

> changes in vaginal discharge
> intestinal cramping with or without diarrhoea
> uterine contractions (these can be felt as a tightening and are not necessarily painful; it is possible for PTL to present without obvious contractions and for the cervix to dilate 'silently').

Complex emotional picture

The psychological consequences of multiple pregnancies can be complicated and challenging, and practitioners need to be aware of the potential for this to be a primary issue and to provide opportunities wherever possible for couples to express their true feelings. For some women, the knowledge that a pregnancy started off with twins but that one of them has been lost and is still being carried can be difficult to accept, and morbid thoughts can haunt the remaining pregnancy, with fears about what will be delivered dominating the pre-birth period. Sensitivity and clear explanations of what to expect can go a long way towards assuaging such anxieties, enabling successful adjustment to occur. The death of a twin *in utero* can lead to enormous difficulties, with emotions shifting between shock and grief and a desperate hope and desire to will the remaining twin to survive. The close proximity of life and death, literally in the same womb, can affect couples profoundly, and it can take them a long time to come to terms with it. The surviving twin can remain unconsciously linked with the loss for some time even after birth.

In MC pregnancies, when parents are made aware of the extra risks posed by the nature of their pregnancy, fear and bewilderment typically accompany the weeks and months of waiting and uncertainty. For some, the regular screening and assessments enable them to prepare themselves for the outcome, whereas for others it can be an unbearably painful time of high anxiety. Maternal bonding may unconsciously be blocked, and the normal process of imaginative introspection that pregnancy represents may be replaced by negative thoughts about what lies ahead. For mothers, worries and feelings of guilt about how they may have contributed to the situation can dominate the psychological landscape throughout the pregnancy, and the difficulties continue when preterm labour abruptly ends the pregnancy. The physical separation from their mothers that is necessary for premature babies mirrors the emotional separation that can occur, as some parents will avoid attachment in case one or more of the babies die.

Parents of a higher-order multiple pregnancy face additional dilemmas, as selective fetal reduction may be advised in order to improve the outcome for the remaining fetuses. This issue is fraught with emotional conflict, and for many the deliberate termination of a life is highly controversial. As most higher-order multiples arise from fertility treatments, the decision to end the life of a longed-for baby can be extremely distressing for couples, and some find it an unbearable burden.

> Following IVF treatment, 42-year-old Rosie was carrying triplets and was advised to undergo selective fetal reduction at 12 weeks. Rosie and her partner received no counselling before the procedure, and struggled with the ethical dilemmas that they faced, independently seeking help from support groups and close family members. Although the couple decided relatively quickly to undergo the reduction, Rosie found the procedure emotionally traumatic, was very disturbed by the screen images of three healthy fetuses, and found the decision to end the life of one of them hard to come to terms with. In the months following the reduction, the pregnancy was fraught with problems and, perhaps understandably, both partners experienced profound feelings of guilt, regret and deep sorrow mingled with high levels of anxiety and fear.

The availability of psychological support and counselling before and after selective fetal reduction is strongly recommended to allow couples to openly discuss their feelings and to reach a position of acceptance. The ethical dilemmas that arise are often impossible for couples to share with others, and they can face months or even years of emotional turmoil if insufficient support is available to them. Emotional exchange between the parents before and after the procedure plays a very important part in the grief process. I always urge couples to seek professional psychological support in these circumstances, even if they do not recognise their need for help at the time, as unresolved emotional conflicts can resurface and cause greater problems later.

INFERTILITY

Although assisted conception has greatly improved the likelihood of infertile couples achieving their families, the use of fertility drugs and technologies is associated with an increased incidence of multiple pregnancies. In addition to the higher risk posed by this, there are particular issues related to infertility that may threaten a pregnancy.

Ovulation induction

Ovulation induction is one of the safest and cheapest means of treating anovulatory infertility, which is the primary abnormality in around 20% of infertile couples. However, all procedures that involve ovarian stimulation will lead to a higher than normal risk of multiple birth. In the UK, the current guidelines of the National Institute for Health and Clinical Excellence (NICE) state that women undergoing treatment with clomifene citrate (Clomid) should be offered ultrasound monitoring to ensure that they receive a dose that minimises this risk.[2] However, in my experience, this guideline is often overlooked, probably due to financial constraints, leading to the situation where a short-term financial saving results in the much greater financial demands posed by the sequelae of multiple pregnancy. In the USA and Europe, multiple pregnancy occurs in 2–13% of women who take clomifene citrate, compared with a spontaneous rate of 1–2% of women.[2] It is established in the literature that although approximately 75% of patients will ovulate following the administration of clomifene, less than 50% of them will conceive, and spontaneous miscarriages occur in about 13–25% of such pregnancies.[7]

Polycystic ovarian syndrome

Polycystic ovarian syndrome (PCOS) accounts for around 75% of anovulatory cases of infertility. Women with PCOS are at increased risk of spontaneous miscarriage. Although the exact pathophysiological mechanism is unclear, the elevated luteinising hormone (LH) level that characterises the syndrome has in the past been thought to be responsible, although recent research suggests this is unlikely. Instead, hyperandrogenaemia, obesity and hyperinsulinaemia have been identified as more probable contributory factors.[8] Clomifene citrate has traditionally been the first-line treatment for women with anovulatory PCOS who wish to conceive. In cases that are resistant to clomifene, and in women who fail to conceive, gonadotrophins may be given. Women with PCOS who are treated with gonadotrophins have a multiple pregnancy rate of 36%. In recent years the use of metformin in PCOS has become increasingly widespread, and there is some evidence to suggest that this may have a number of protective effects in pregnancy by reducing complications such as gestational diabetes and early pregnancy loss.[9]

IVF

Although some studies have identified a higher incidence of miscarriage among women who conceive through IVF (and other assisted conception methods) compared with that in the general population, accurate comparisons are problematic, as assisted pregnancies are under intense scrutiny, and very early losses are noted at a stage when they may normally go unrecognised. Limited data exist for understanding the risks according to different maternal ages, ART procedures, gestational stage, and so on, and at the present time the question of whether ART pregnancies carry a higher risk of loss remains unanswered.[3] Perhaps the most important factor underlying any apparent increased risk of miscarriage in this group is maternal age, as women undergoing ART tend to be older, and also many of them have experienced previous losses, both of which are known risk factors for spontaneous miscarriage. However, evidence from studies that have controlled for these factors does show that the risk of miscarriage is significantly higher than that for natural conceptions, and that some treatment-specific factors may contribute to this, such as higher levels of ovarian stimulation.[10]

Although the goal of IVF is to maximise the likelihood of a successful pregnancy while minimising the risk of multiple birth, the number of multiples arising from IVF remains a concern. The majority of twin pregnancies following IVF are dizygotic, due to the transfer of more than one embryo, but it is estimated that there is a twofold increase in the incidence of monozygotic twins following IVF. A recent meta-analysis confirmed that there is a 2.25-fold higher risk following IVF than in natural conception, plus an apparently higher risk with some ART techniques, such as intracytoplasmic sperm injection (ICSI) and blastocyst transfer.[11]

Despite awareness among healthcare professionals of the need to reduce the number of multiple births, and moves in some countries towards single embryo transfer, patient acceptance of this is far from routine. Surveys have suggested that the prospect of multiple pregnancies is not necessarily viewed as an adverse outcome by patients who are facing infertility treatment.[2] In my practice it is commonplace for couples undergoing IVF treatment to react negatively if their doctor advises single embryo transfer. Despite a broad awareness of the practical difficulties of coping with twins, my patients often tend to gloss over these and see twins as a welcome end to their fertility journeys, which are frequently self-funded and financially, physically and psychologically demanding. It is rare for patients to engage with information on the medical implications of multiple pregnancies for themselves or their babies. Improved guidance from the fertility clinics on this topic would be welcome.

> Carolyn successfully underwent IVF two years ago, and gave birth to twin boys. Wishing to enlarge their family to three, the couple embarked upon further IVF treatment, and discussions between Carolyn and her husband centred on the dilemma of how many embryos they would have replaced. Gambling that as they had already had a successful twin pregnancy, this would surely be unlikely to happen twice, on the day of embryo transfer they decided against single embryo transfer, opting instead to have two embryos replaced and hoping that only one would implant. The treatment was successful, at the first scan two heartbeats were detected, and at the time of writing Carolyn's second twin pregnancy is moving into its third trimester.

Ectopic pregnancy

An ectopic pregnancy is one that implants outside the uterine cavity, and it represents a form of early pregnancy loss. In recent decades the incidence of ectopic pregnancy has increased substantially. This may be due to a number of risk factors (*see* Box 3.2), as well as to earlier detection due to improved screening. Ectopic pregnancies occur in 3–5% of ART cycles. Despite the fact that embryos are transferred into the uterine cavity in IVF, it is thought that uterine contractions may facilitate movement into the Fallopian tubes, with the majority returning to the uterine cavity.[1]

BOX 3.2: Risk factors for ectopic pregnancy

- Chlamydia infection
- Current intrauterine device
- Endometriosis
- History of infertility
- Increased maternal age
- Pelvic inflammatory disease
- Previous ectopic pregnancy

- Previous peritonitis or pelvic surgery (e.g. appendicitis)
- Previous tubal surgery (e.g. failed sterilisation or reversal of sterilisation)
- Smoking

Ectopic pregnancy can have long-term implications and serious consequences, especially if diagnosis and treatment are delayed. Indeed, depending on several factors, even when surgical treatment is prompt, the removal of part or all of the woman's Fallopian tube (in tubal ectopics) may be necessary. For a woman, this can mean having to face recovery not only from surgery, but also from losing the pregnancy and an important aspect of her feminine self. For some women this presents major worries and doubts about their future ability to achieve their family, which can persist long after physical healing has occurred.

Mary and her husband had been trying to conceive for 3 years, and after undergoing extensive investigations that led to a diagnosis of unexplained infertility, they were advised that IVF would be their best option. They did not feel quite ready to accept that this was the path for them, and as Mary was only 29 years of age, they believed that they could afford to wait a little longer before, as they saw it, 'giving up' on their natural fertility. After a further few months Mary duly conceived naturally, only for her immense joy to be crushed when it was discovered that the pregnancy was ectopic. After surgery to remove her left Fallopian tube, Mary was devastated to be told that her remaining tube was damaged to the extent that natural conception was highly unlikely, and that if she underwent IVF, removal of the remaining tube first would be best to avoid the risk of further ectopic pregnancies. Mary's emotional recovery took many months as she was consumed by distress about what she had lost. Her self-esteem plummeted and she felt an overwhelming sense of failure. She described her feelings as veering between anger and profound grief. Her anger was directed both at herself and her 'failed' body, and at her doctor, who had delivered the news in a way that she found cold, uncaring and too matter-of-fact. She grieved both for her lost pregnancy and for her own fertility.

REFERENCES

1 Edmonds DK. *Dewhurst's Textbook of Obstetrics and Gynaecology.* 7th edn. Oxford: Blackwell Publishing; 2007.

2 National Institute for Health and Clinical Excellence (NICE). *Fertility Assessment and Treatment for People with Fertility Problems: CG11.* London: NICE; 2004. www.nice.org.uk/CG011 (accessed 10 October 2010).

3 Farr SL, Schieve L, Jamieson DJ. Pregnancy loss among pregnancies conceived through assisted reproductive technology, United States, 1999–2002. *American Journal of Epidemiology* 2007; **165**: 1380–88.

4 James DK, Steer PJ, Weiner CP *et al. High Risk Pregnancy Management Options.* 3rd edn. Philadelphia, PA: Elsevier; 2006.

5 Norwitz E, Schorge J. *Obstetrics and Gynaecology at a Glance.* 2nd edn. Malden, MA: Blackwell Publishing Inc; 2006.

6 Gilbert E, Harmon J. *Manual of High Risk Pregnancy and Delivery.* 3rd edn. St Louis, MO: Mosby; 2003.

7 Ballian N, Mantoudis E, Kaltsas G. Pregnancy following ovarian drilling in a woman with polycystic ovary syndrome and nine previous first trimester miscarriages. *Archives of Gynecology and Obstetrics* 2006; **273**: 384–6.

8 Cocksedge K, Saravelos S, Wang Q *et al.* Does free androgen index predict subsequent pregnancy outcome in women with recurrent miscarriage? *Human Reproduction* 2008; **23**: 797–802.

9 Fleming R, Sattar N. Should patients with polycystic ovary syndrome be treated with metformin? In: Allahbadia G, Agrawal R, eds. *Polycystic Ovary Syndrome.* Tunbridge Wells: Anshan; 2007.

10 Wang JX, Norman RJ, Wilcox AJ. Incidence of spontaneous abortion among pregnancies produced by assisted reproductive technology. *Human Reproduction* 2004; **19**: 272–7.

11 Vitthala S, Gelbaya TA, Brison D *et al.* The risk of monozygotic twins after assisted reproductive technology: a systematic review and meta-analysis. *Human Reproduction Update* 2009; **15**: 45–55.

CHAPTER 4

Investigations, treatment and management

INTRODUCTION

Some women recover from one miscarriage within a relatively short time period, and they remain optimistic about a future pregnancy. Far fewer women remain as optimistic following a second or third loss, as worries mount over whether a successful pregnancy will ever happen. A preoccupation with trying to become pregnant and staying pregnant can eventually dominate the lives of women and their partners. The need to find out the reason why their pregnancies fail can be overwhelming, and many will fear that there is something fundamentally wrong with them which, until it is fixed, will forever blight their hopes of achieving their desired family. In the case of stillbirth, many parents want to know as much as possible about why their baby died, not least in order to protect themselves from such a distressing event occurring again.

With the high number of possible causes and unknown factors involved in pregnancy loss, the issue of when to investigate and which tests and treatments to offer is surrounded by a notable degree of professional controversy. Women are exposed to conflicting and varying information. This chapter covers the options that are currently available for investigating the causes, the conventional management of pregnancy loss, and treatments that may be offered to prevent it from happening again. It must be emphasised that some of these will not always be available, while others are considered by many clinicians to be experimental and unproven.

MANAGEMENT AND TREATMENT OF EARLY PREGNANCY FAILURE

The introduction of Early Pregnancy Units (EPUs) in hospitals in recent years means that patients and professionals have a dedicated unit through which women can be sensitively diagnosed and supported when things appear to be going wrong. The NHS has more than 250 EPUs across the UK. They are often found in dedicated areas within gynaecology units and staffed by a multi-disciplinary team of doctors, nurses, ultrasonographers, midwives and support staff. Women should go to their local EPU in the following circumstances:[1]

> if bleeding occurs during the first 13 weeks of pregnancy
> if abdominal, pelvic or back pain is experienced during the first 13 weeks of pregnancy
> if they are being constantly sick
> if they suspect for any reason at all that they might be having a miscarriage
> if they are referred by their GP or practice nurse, consultant or midwife, which may be because they have had a previous ectopic pregnancy, two or more miscarriages, previous tubal surgery or an intrauterine contraceptive device *in situ*.

In some localities women can self-refer to EPUs, while in others a GP or midwife referral may be required. At the unit, the woman's history will be taken, her blood and urine may be tested, and a transvaginal ultrasound scan may be performed to check on the development of the pregnancy. It may be necessary for the woman to have a physical examination to assess the cervix. Depending on the findings of all these steps, a plan of management will be prepared. Follow-up arrangements should be in place before the woman leaves the unit, and written advice and contact telephone numbers should be provided.[1]

Miscarriage

The most common complication seen in early pregnancy is miscarriage. The vast majority of miscarriages occur early, before 12 weeks' gestation, and vaginal bleeding is the most common presenting symptom, often accompanied by cramping, central, low abdominal pain. However, some women will not be aware of any problem with their pregnancy until their first scan.

Not all bleeding in early pregnancy signifies miscarriage, but it should always be reported and the woman should be examined. If the cervical os is open, the pregnancy is failing and miscarriage is inevitable. However, if the os is closed, a transvaginal ultrasound scan will reveal whether the fetus is viable or not. Depending on the diagnosis (*see* Box 4.1), different options may be offered.

BOX 4.1: Types of miscarriage

Threatened
Bleeding before 24 weeks with a closed cervical os and confirmed viable fetus

Inevitable
Bleeding before 24 weeks with an open cervical os

Missed/delayed/silent
Scan shows intrauterine fetal demise, the cervix is closed and there is complete retention of products of conception. Bleeding may or may not have occurred

Incomplete
Scan shows partial or imminent expulsion of products of conception through open cervix

Complete
Scan shows complete expulsion of products of conception, and the cervix is closed

---

Management of miscarriage

Although the uterus will eventually expel the products of conception when a fetus dies, this can take several weeks, and traditionally the risk of infection meant that surgical evacuation of the uterus was standard treatment. Known colloquially as a 'D&C', but more correctly as an evacuation of retained products of conception (ERPC), this is a quick and straightforward procedure that is performed under general anaesthetic in the UK. In recent years expectant and medical management options have developed, which offer welcome choices for those who wish to avoid undergoing a surgical procedure. Studies have shown that there is no difference in infection rates between expectant and surgical options, although surgery remains the treatment of choice if bleeding is severe or infection is present.

Expectant management is usually what will be advised in general practice for complete and some cases of incomplete miscarriage, and it is estimated that 74% of non-viable pregnancies do not require any intervention.[2] However, unless women are carefully and sensitively advised about what to expect and they feel confident about the decision, this option can be interpreted as them being put aside or the miscarriage not being taken seriously, whereas in fact the body is being allowed time to work naturally without the need for recourse to unnecessary medical procedures.[3] Good communication is essential to allow this option to be fully appreciated. Medical management involves the administration either orally or vaginally of pharmaceuticals to ensure full evacuation of retained tissue, and although it is offered as an outpatient procedure in some areas, the degree of pain that is experienced can require analgesia. It is an option in some cases of silent and incomplete miscarriage.

Every miscarriage is different. It can be a very frightening event, especially if the woman has not previously experienced a miscarriage. On the whole, healthcare professionals are not always very good at preparing women for this event.[3,4] Studies on women's experiences of miscarriage management highlight the importance of women and their partners receiving appropriate information about the management options available to them, and having their views taken into consideration when the choice of treatment is made.[4] For some women, there is a sense that a surgical procedure ends the pregnancy properly, and it can be a welcome marking of this, whereas for others it is an unwelcome intervention that removes the choice of allowing their body to end the pregnancy. Clearly it is impossible to satisfy the needs of everyone, but themes that persistently emerge in studies of women's experiences are that poor communication and a perceived lack of empathy among medical staff lead to more negative experiences for women. Clear and sensitively delivered information about the degree of pain and bleeding that may be expected is an example of where a small change in information availability could lead to major improvements in women's experiences.

Investigation and treatment of recurrent miscarriage
Reproductive immune testing

Reproductive immunology is an area of research and treatment that, with the exception of screening for and treatment of antiphospholipid antibodies (aPL) (which is discussed here separately), attracts much debate and controversy. Offered by a few fertility clinics and reproductive clinicians in the UK to women who have experienced previous IVF failure or recurrent miscarriage, the majority of the tests and treatments involved are relatively new. At the time of writing, the results of the few clinical trials that have been conducted in this field remain unreliable and contradictory, characterised by small sample sizes and many confounding variables.

Testing typically involves blood tests to measure the levels of natural killer (NK) cells and their activity. However, there are differences between NK cells in peripheral blood and those found in the uterine environment (uNK cells), and some experts question the relevance and reliability of using information from blood samples. Disagreement focuses on the following areas.

➤ There are phenotypic and functional differences between NK cells in peripheral blood and those in the uterine environment.
➤ uNK cells are not found in the peripheral blood.
➤ The reliability of extrapolating from a blood sample to what is occurring at the maternal–fetal interface is questionable.
➤ Peripheral NK cells are subject to a number of variables, including parity of the mother.
➤ There is no agreed value that constitutes a raised NK cell level.
➤ No association between uNK cell number and function has been demonstrated.
➤ There is no evidence that uNK cells are destructive and attack placental, embryonic or fetal cells.

However, despite the debate and lack of scientific agreement, treatments to suppress NK cells are given by those doctors who adopt this approach if raised levels are identified (*see* Box 4.2). It is notable that these treatments are not licensed for use in reproductive medicine, and therefore many doctors question their integration at the present time into clinical practice outside the controlled environment of a research trial.

BOX 4.2: Treatments given for reproductive immune problems

Glucocorticoids (steroids) Given to suppress immune responses. Concerns over safety in pregnancy: the UK Committee on Safety of Medicines advises that there is a small risk of poor fetal growth, preterm birth, pre-eclampsia and gestational diabetes linked with use of this treatment.[5] Trials with IVF patients have shown no increase in live birth rate with steroid use[6]

Intravenous immunoglobulin (IVIg) Immunotherapy given to promote immune tolerance of the fetus. Made up of antibodies from blood plasma of multiple donors, administered by intravenous drip. Small trials with inadequate rigour have shown beneficial results in preventing miscarriage, but larger studies are lacking, and the systematic reviews that exist refute the evidence that IVIg improves live birth rates in RM.[7-9] Very expensive

Anti-TNF-α agents TNF-α blocking agents stop inflammation and reduce the body's ability to fight infection. Enoval, Remicade and Humira are used by some clinics that offer immunotherapy; all of them have potentially serious side-effects, and the *British National Formulary* states that Remicade should not be used in pregnancy. The effects of Humira on reproduction and fetal growth are not known

Aspirin and heparin Given to women with antiphospholipid syndrome, aspirin is started as soon as pregnancy is confirmed, and heparin is started once the fetal heartbeat is detected (around 6.5 weeks). Treatment stops at 34 weeks. Trials have confirmed effectiveness in cases of RM due to antiphospolipid syndrome,[10] but the benefits of similar treatment for RM in women with thrombophilias remain unproven

The Royal College of Obstetricians and Gynaecologists (RCOG) Opinion Paper[11] published in 2008 states:

> With the exception of aPL testing among women with recurrent miscarriage, there is little evidence to support any particular test or immunomodulatory treatment in the investigation and treatment of couples with reproductive failure. These tests and treatments should be restricted to those entered into formal research studies.

However, there are many doctors working in the field, for whose patients such treatment appears to lead to successful pregnancies, who disagree with this position despite the lack of scientific evidence. Because treatment seems to offer hope for some women, and high-profile media coverage of 'miracle' babies resulting from these treatments raises awareness of their availability, some women understandably want to pursue this route. In my clinic I see increasing numbers of women each year who actively seek out doctors and clinics that will treat them for immunological reasons, even if they are advised against this by other doctors who are equally eminent in the field. It is not within my remit as a practitioner of complementary medicine to offer advice to my patients on this controversial area, but I do urge them to make sure that they know the possible risks as well as the benefits of any tests or treatments they are offered, not least in view of the high financial costs currently associated with these. A thorough discussion with their doctor before embarking on any tests should provide them with clear and acceptable explanations as to why the tests and/or treatments are being recommended, what they will involve, and a frank assessment of the benefits and the possible side-effects and risks. Only after this will the patient be fully able to consider whether this avenue is right for them.

Antiphospholipid syndrome (APS)

Antiphospholipid syndrome is an example of an autoimmune-mediated pregnancy loss that in recent years has emerged as one of the most important treatable causes of recurrent implantation failure and RM. It is diagnosed if a woman tests positive for antiphospholipid antibodies (aPL) on two separate occasions 6 weeks apart, together with one or more of the following:

➤ previous thrombosis
➤ one or more unexplained pregnancy losses
➤ one or more premature births
➤ intrauterine growth restriction in a previous pregnancy
➤ pre-eclampsia.

Once diagnosed, women are usually advised to start treatment (*see* Box 4.2) as soon as they become pregnant, or in some cases before that. In general, treatment for APS has a high success rate, but for some unfortunate women treatment will fail, or they may miscarry for reasons unconnected with the condition, such as chromosomal problems. Additional psychological support is very important in these cases, as following a diagnosis of APS great optimism and relief that their problems are behind them often accompany couples into the next pregnancy.

Screening for chromosomal problems

More females than males are affected by structural chromosomal abnormalities, and for these to cause RM, one partner must have a chromosomal abnormality or produce recurrent abnormalities in the embryo (e.g. through increasing maternal age). The most common karyotypic abnormality found in parental chromosomal screening is a balanced or reciprocal translocation. Fetal aneuploidy is the most common cause of miscarriage and is mostly related to maternal age. Where screening detects abnormalities, genetic counselling that explores the couple's individual prognosis should be offered.

Some couples may decide to undergo IVF with pre-implantation genetic diagnosis (PGD). This screens embryos in order to obtain a genetic diagnosis, only replacing into the uterus those that are normal. As only unaffected embryos are replaced, PGD offers couples who are affected by karyotypic abnormalities the opportunity to avoid having to decide whether to terminate a viable pregnancy. However, the following points should be noted.

➤ PGD is only available on embryos created through IVF.
➤ IVF is costly as well as physically and psychologically challenging for couples.
➤ The live birth rate for those with reciprocal translocation who conceive naturally, even after three miscarriages, is around 50–65%, compared with 29–38% for each IVF cycle in similar patients.[2]

Other options are to use donor sperm or eggs in IVF treatment or to undergo prenatal diagnosis. However, by that stage no treatment will be available if abnormalities are detected, and the parents then have to face the decision to terminate the pregnancy, a distressing decision that in most cases will be made during the second trimester.

Additional investigations

Although maternal screening for endocrine disorders has traditionally been undertaken, the prevalence of these disorders does not appear to be higher in women with RM than in the general population, and is not considered as valuable as was once thought.[11] However, diagnosis and treatment of underlying disease are required as, if left untreated or poorly controlled, this is likely to contribute to RM (in addition to other problems associated with untreated disease).

Where luteal phase defect may be thought to be the cause of recurrent losses, progesterone supplementation is commonly prescribed, although its therapeutic benefit is based upon speculation and is not supported by clinical evidence.[12] In cases of polycystic ovary syndrome (PCOS), attention has previously focused on suppression of luteinising hormone. However, clinical trial results demonstrated no reduction in miscarriage rates. Attention is now focusing on the role that insulin resistance plays in pregnancy loss and PCOS. Recently the insulin-sensitising drug metformin has attracted interest, and studies have demonstrated that it improves pregnancy outcome.[13,14] This is thought to be due to metformin leading to improvements in the uterine environment and possibly better egg quality.[15]

Ectopic pregnancy

This is suspected in cases where there is a positive pregnancy test, bleeding and/or pain, and a transvaginal ultrasound scan reveals an empty uterus. In a few cases, the situation will be a medical emergency that requires immediate surgery. Surgical management is usually via either laparotomy or laparoscopy to remove the ectopic and affected structures. Conservation of the Fallopian tubes is attempted wherever possible. Medical management has been introduced for certain cases, but with limited availability, in a few hospitals.

Gestational trophoblastic disease

Complete moles typically cause abnormal vaginal bleeding in the first trimester, whereas partial moles usually present as a missed miscarriage during the first or early second trimester. Most cases will only be diagnosed following an ERPC for a missed miscarriage, and histological findings reveal the mole. Although gestational trophoblastic disease is a very rare complication, some cases can become malignant, and follow-up care is important in all cases. Women are followed up for 6 months following the diagnosis, and in the very unlikely event of malignancy, chemotherapy will be offered.

THE VALUE OF SUPPORTIVE CARE

For many of the women whom I see, feelings of frustration arise when they have experienced a miscarriage and are then told that they have to wait until the third miscarriage before any testing can be undertaken. Such feelings of frustration are understandable, especially if we bear in mind that they have visited their doctor in the aftermath of a loss of life. It is difficult to envisage other circumstances that would result in a life being lost before investigations could be started. That being said, miscarriage is common, and even if a problem is discovered, in many cases not much can be done about it and most women will eventually successfully become pregnant without any intervention. Nevertheless, healthcare professionals should recognise the need for women to ask questions and to seek explanations, and even if they do not have all the answers, they should strive at all times to adopt a supportive and caring attitude towards women both during and after the trauma of miscarriage. Good communication can prevent women from feeling, as they commonly report, that their experience has been quickly dismissed or, worse, belittled.

SECOND- AND THIRD-TRIMESTER LOSS

In some cases of pregnancy loss there is overlap through the trimesters. For example, APS causes problems in early and late pregnancy, so in some respects the distinction that is made in this section is unnecessary. However, for reasons of clarity, there are a few specific topics which are discussed here.

Preterm labour

Defined in the UK as labour occurring after 24 weeks' and before 37 weeks' gestation, the incidence of preterm labour (PTL) is rising. It can occur spontaneously and unexpectedly, or it may be medically induced (e.g. in order to address severe fetal intrauterine growth retardation, or in the interests of the mother's health). Prevention and treatment of spontaneous PTL is difficult, and involves seeking to identify those women who are at risk (*see* Chapter 3), and stopping contractions in women who are already in established labour. For women in their first pregnancy there is currently no reliable method for predicting PTL, but if there is a history of a previous preterm delivery there is a high risk of this recurring in future pregnancies. Although, medically speaking, late miscarriage and PTL are quite distinct, for parents the experience of both is very similar and involves high levels of fear and distress. This is significantly alleviated if a clear understanding is shown of the parents' distress by those around them and honest compassion is demonstrated.

Cervical cerclage
It is thought that there are probably several similarities between the events that cause second-trimester loss and PTL that involve cervical incompetence. In women with any of the following, transvaginal ultrasound measurement of cervical length can be used to help to predict those at risk:
➤ history of cervical surgery or trauma
➤ previous rapid or relatively painless second-trimester loss
➤ previous relatively rapid or painless PTL
➤ congenital cervical hypoplasia.

Ideally, measurements are taken serially during the second and early third trimesters, although a single measurement in the second trimester is sometimes offered. Cervical cerclage, which involves the insertion of a stitch, or suture, is the mainstay of treatment of cervical incompetence, and is performed either at around 12–14 weeks or later as an emergency measure. Debate over whether prophylactic cervical cerclage has real benefits for the majority of women who undergo the procedure is ongoing. It is known that for every 25 cerclages that are inserted, one woman will benefit. The procedure is not without risk, and is performed either transvaginally or (less commonly) transabdominally. In both cases the patient is required to have complete rest during recovery, which takes several weeks. Undoubtedly some women undergo what is quite a major intervention unnecessarily, but on the other hand the procedure serves a real purpose in reassuring women that their pregnancy will continue successfully, and the psychological benefits of this alone can be immense.

The use of drugs to prevent preterm labour
Studies published in recent years have indicated a beneficial role for progesterone supplementation from weeks 16–36 in preventing PTL in women at risk, and there are few if any side-effects associated with its use.[16] Other drugs are used to delay contractions in acute PTL, but they have limited benefit, carry a number of risks and are not used prophylactically.

Stillbirth and intrauterine death

Loss of a pregnancy after 24 weeks in the UK is termed intrauterine death, which when delivered is a stillbirth. It can occur without warning or it may be anticipated and prepared for. When an intrauterine death has been confirmed, some parents do not want to delay the induction of labour, while others prefer to be given time to come to terms with the diagnosis and make both practical and emotional preparations. Once started, the process of induction and labour can take several days to complete and may be especially difficult for both parents and staff. The sensitivity with which the parents are cared for throughout this time has lasting implications for their recovery through the subsequent grieving process.[17]

In some cases, the parents will have decided to continue with the pregnancy in the knowledge that the baby will not survive. This may be for a number of reasons:

➤ late diagnosis of abnormality may have meant that a termination was not acceptable to them
➤ religious or ethical objections to termination may have removed this option for them
➤ a desire to plan and prepare for the birth and death of their baby
➤ the opportunity to spend time, however short, with their baby after birth
➤ inability to accept the diagnosis.

Carefully coordinated management of such cases is important to ensure that the parents' wishes are respected and that no unnecessary stress and emotional disturbance are created for them. Continuity of care and support from those involved in looking after the mother is important, and it helps to ease the bewildering sense of isolation that is reported by many couples. It can be agonising for women in this situation to be seen in routine antenatal settings where they will wait with others whose pregnancies are progressing normally, or to be seen by different staff every time. Sensitivity and excellent communication between staff are essential in order to minimise the distress caused by the situation.

Multiple pregnancy

Issues in multiple pregnancy are often highly complex, and are made more or less so by the chorionicity of the pregnancy (*see* Chapter 3). For example, multiplets are especially prone to discordant growth, and the expectant management of this must be balanced against the risk of unnecessarily causing premature delivery by early intervention. In other words, it must be decided whether early induced delivery to save an affected baby is the right course of action when it leads to the unaffected baby being born earlier than necessary. In multiple pregnancies, one baby may die *in utero* but the pregnancy continues with the surviving babies, or the parents may be offered selective feticide if one of the babies has a serious abnormality. This is an unthinkable option for many parents when it is first offered. In all cases of intrauterine death, increased monitoring of the survivor is standard care, but levels of parental anxiety about the possibility that the dead baby will harm the survivor can be overwhelmingly high. Some parents will wish to see the lost baby on ultrasound scans and after birth. These wishes should be respected, as this can greatly assist the process of mourning and recovery. Parents in these situations will experience tremendous emotional turmoil, and require sensitivity, genuine understanding and compassion from everyone involved in their case.

REFERENCES

1 www.earlypregnancy.org.uk/default.asp

2 Edmonds DK. *Dewhurst's Textbook of Obstetrics and Gynaecology.* 7th edn. Oxford: Blackwell Publishing; 2007.

3 Moulder C. *Miscarriage: women's experiences and needs.* London: Routledge; 2001.

4 Smith LF, Frost J, Levitas R *et al.* Women's experiences of three early miscarriage management options: a qualitative study. *British Journal of General Practice* 2006; **56**: 198–205.

5 Laskin CA, Bombardier C, Hannah ME *et al.* Prednisone and aspirin in women with autoantibodies and unexplained fetal loss. *New England Journal of Medicine* 1997; **337**: 148–53.

6 Boomsma CM, Keay SD, Macklon NS. Peri-implantation glucocorticoid administration for assisted reproductive technology cycles. *Cochrane Database of Systematic Reviews* 2007; **1**: CD005996.

7 Hutton B, Sharma R, Fergusson D *et al.* Use of intravenous immunoglobulin for treatment of recurrent miscarriage: a systematic review. *British Journal of Obstetrics and Gynaecology* 2007; **114**: 134–42.

8 Porter TF, La Coursiere Y, Scott JR. Immunotherapy for recurrent miscarriage. *Cochrane Database of Systematic Reviews* 2006; **19(2)**: CD000112.

9 Scott JR. Immunotherapy for recurrent miscarriage. *Cochrane Database of Systematic Reviews* 2003; **1**: CD000112.

10 Empson M, Lassere M, Craig JC *et al*. Recurrent pregnancy loss with antiphospholipid antibody: a systematic review of therapeutic trials. *Obstetrics and Gynecology* 2002; **99**: 135–44.

11 Royal College of Obstetricians and Gynaecologists. *The Investigation and Treatment of Recurrent Miscarriage. Guideline No. 17.* London: RCOG Press; 2003.

12 Oates-Whitehead RM, Haas DM, Carrrier JA. Progestogen for preventing miscarriage. *Cochrane Database of Systematic Reviews* 2003; **4**: CD003511.

13 Ballian N, Mantoudis E, Kaltsas G. Pregnancy following ovarian drilling in a woman with polycystic ovary syndrome and nine previous first trimester miscarriages. *Archives of Gynecology and Obstetrics* 2006; **273**: 384–6.

14 Glueck CJ, Wang P, Goldenberg N *et al*. Pregnancy outcomes among women with polycystic ovary syndrome treated with metformin. *Human Reproduction* 2002; **17**: 2858–64.

15 Ruvalcaba L, Cubillos S, Bermúdez A *et al*. Glucose intolerance in the polycystic ovary syndrome: role of pancreatic beta-cell. In: Allahbadia G, Agrawal R, eds. *Polycystic Ovary Syndrome*. Tunbridge Wells: Anshan; 2007.

16 Dodd JM, Flenady V, Cincotta R *et al*. Prenatal administration of progesterone for preventing preterm birth in women considered to be at risk of preterm birth. *Cochrane Database of Systematic Reviews* 2006; **1**: CD004947.

17 Schott J, Henley A, Kohner N. *Pregnancy Loss and the Death of a Baby: guidelines for professionals*. 3rd edn. London: Sands; 2007.

CHAPTER 5

Psychological issues in pregnancy loss

INTRODUCTION

Despite being a common occurrence and not usually considered a major medical event, miscarriage is far from insignificant for the individuals involved. Death in later life is accompanied by recognised social rituals, whereas these are lacking in pregnancy loss, and people often do not know what to say or do or how to react to those involved. It is only in recent years that the impact of such loss has received greater attention, largely through the work of groups such as the Miscarriage Association (MA) and the Stillbirth and Neonatal Death Society (SANDS). However, despite improved general awareness among the public and healthcare professionals of the emotional significance of pregnancy loss, this is not always reflected in the attitudes that are adopted towards women who are undergoing the highly personal and complex emotional crisis that pregnancy loss represents.[1,2] Careless and casual comments, lack of sensitivity to the situation, or a general attempt to minimise emotional distress (e.g. in early-trimester losses by talking about cells and tissue rather than babies) are reported by women, and only serve to emphasise the isolation of their grief.

WHEN DOES LOSS BECOME DEATH?
Perceptions of loss

It is all too common for people who have never experienced a miscarriage to dismiss or minimise the experiences of those who do experience it. There is no neatly defined stage of pregnancy at which women are devastated by the ending of it. For some women, profound attachment to their pregnancy begins before conception, and an early miscarriage can be deeply traumatic, whereas for others the pregnancy does not become real until the baby is born. What is important is that every loss has unique significance to those involved, and many women simply wish to have this acknowledged, but in society as a whole and in medicine generally this is not always the case.

Lack of recognition of the loss as a baby

The procedures that occur following a miscarriage and the terminology used by healthcare professionals when referring to these procedures can have psychological consequences that affect the ability of some women to mourn and recover from early miscarriage. Whereas professionals commonly refer to 'products of conception', women often identify their loss with a baby. The lack of social or medical recognition that the loss was a baby compounds the isolation that is felt by many women, and can leave them grappling with difficult emotional reactions long after physical recovery has taken place.[3] Recent technological advances mean that women can identify with their pregnancy very early on, and this early identification may well exacerbate the difficulties of adjusting to an early pregnancy loss.

> Philippa, a paediatric nurse, started bleeding heavily 5 days after discovering that she was pregnant. Highly anxious and concerned about the amount of bleeding, she visited her GP 5 days later, when the bleeding was still continuing. She was sent home after being told that she was 'just having a late period' and that it was too early to really view what was happening to her as a miscarriage and the bleeding was a normal period. She recounted this to me 4 years after the event and her anger was still very palpable. Despite knowing that medically her experience was common, and not that interesting or important, her GP's dismissal of her and her loss added to her distress.

In surveys, the emotional impact of miscarriage is often cited as an area that receives little wider recognition. In one study, over 94% of parents felt that they were grieving parents who had suffered a genuine loss.[4] The assumption by others either that mourning is not necessary or that it is inappropriate can make adjustment to the loss extremely difficult. This is further complicated by differences in our use of language, along with varying legal, medical and religious definitions of when the loss of a fetus or embryo becomes the death of a baby. Whereas some research in the field points to the majority of parents viewing miscarriage as the loss of a 'real' baby,[4] others make it clear that not all parents relate to their lost pregnancies in this way, perhaps as an attempt to protect themselves from the devastating impact that such a definition may have for them.[1] It is advisable that people avoid defining the event for those involved, and instead go along with however the parents define it themselves, and respect whatever individual meanings and significance it holds for them.

Gestational age is no marker of depth of trauma

A common assumption is that the degree of psychological distress will be proportional to the stage of pregnancy at which loss occurs. However, this is not reflected in several studies, some of which have reported that the intensity of grief following a miscarriage may be as great as that following stillbirth or neonatal death.[3,4] Furthermore, the presence of other children, maternal age, and the number of previous miscarriages that the parents may have experienced are commonly assumed to have a uniform impact on the intensity of emotional response. However, this is not supported by the findings of many researchers.[5-7]

The silent agony

Whereas the trauma of stillbirth is apparent to most, the silent agony of intrauterine death of a twin is less obvious. In multiple pregnancies, one baby may die *in utero* while the remaining baby or babies survive, leading to a complicated parental psychological situation at the time of birth, when intense grief is juxtaposed with relief and joy. At the same time, well-meaning friends and family may urge the parents to ignore the lost baby and celebrate the living one(s).[8]

UNDERSTANDING THE EXPERIENCE

There is considerable evidence that pregnancy loss has a huge impact on the lives of those whom it affects, which can lead to negative psychological reactions for months afterwards, including grief, depression, anger, anxiety and confusion, and some individuals will develop chronic psychiatric morbidity.[5,6] There is not only the actual death of the baby to cope with, but also the loss of hope and joy that this may have represented. However, we should be aware that not everyone will experience such powerful reactions, and some women may experience minimal emotional disturbance.

Every loss is different

Every loss is unique and carries individual significance, but the following factors commonly influence the way in which people react to their pregnancy loss.

Previous obstetric history

A history of recurrent loss may make pregnancy loss increasingly hard to bear, even if it is anticipated, and even more so if treatment has been tried. However far in the past it occurred, guilt, shame or self-recrimination about a previous termination can resurface when another loss occurs.

Fertility issues

Difficulties with conception can make the death of a longed-for baby especially distressing, as the possibility that this may be the last chance of achieving pregnancy can be devastating. Feelings about the loss may be influenced by whether the pregnancy occurred naturally or with assistance, as obstacles to conceiving again (whether financial, medical or emotional) can heighten the distress. Although well-meaning, comments such as 'Well, you can always try again' may be particularly painful to hear and have added poignancy.

Questions about viability

If there are concerns about the viability of the pregnancy, with worrying symptoms and inconclusive findings from scans and tests, the eventual ending of the pregnancy can bring relief. Conversely, guilt and shame may dominate the emotional picture if the woman blames her own negative thoughts for bringing about the end of the pregnancy, or if a couple decide to have a termination.

Maternal age

Older women are likely to be aware of the inherent problems with regard to conceiving again, and the increased risk of miscarriage or fetal abnormalities, and may blame themselves disproportionately when things go wrong.

Interpersonal relationships

If the baby was seen as crucial to the survival of the parental relationship, the loss can have far-reaching consequences. Relationship problems that may have already been present can erupt in the face of blame or hostility. Conversely, some psychosocial studies have shown that for many couples the experience of loss brings them closer together.[4]

Religious and cultural backgrounds

There are those for whom a religious faith can be a source of comfort, whereas for others the devastation of loss may cause them to doubt their faith or to feel anger that such a tragedy occurred.

Social support

The presence or absence of emotionally supportive people either during the experience of loss or in the weeks or months that follow it can alleviate or exacerbate the feelings of failure, guilt and depression that arise. On the other hand, although many well-meaning friends may attempt to provide a degree of support, sometimes their comments can be hurtful or careless and worsen the emotional trauma.

The response of medical professionals

The profound emotional reactions that characterise pregnancy loss can lead to an unwillingness or inability among some medical professionals to engage in this area of a woman's care. In some cases the focusing of effort on the physical management of the event may lead to an unconscious neglect of the emotional issues. In a society where medicine is expected to have the answers and remarkable things can be done to prevent death, it can be difficult for those caring for women who lose their babies to know how to respond, and they may react by emotionally distancing themselves,[8] thus appearing aloof or uncaring. The separation of physical and emotional care at this time is something that is overwhelmingly condemned by those affected by pregnancy loss, whereas expressions of warmth, openness and sorrow offered by medical staff are consistently recognised as making a terrible experience more bearable.[1,8] What parents undoubtedly want is a sense of connection with those who are caring for them.

Expressions and experiences of grief

Although there are cross-cultural differences in the way in which we express grief, a deep and painful sense of loss is almost certainly universal.[9] The initial grief reaction can vary widely, and may include shock, disbelief, and a sense of unreality, guilt, blame, anger and hostility. There are several models of grief which can help us to understand the emotional dynamics that parents may experience, but it is important to recognise that their responses may not always fit neatly into such models.

The process of mourning

Worden[10] describes four tasks of mourning, which have been given context by Jodi Shaefer.[9]

➤ First, it is necessary to intellectually and emotionally accept the reality of the loss. For most people, intellectual acceptance comes well before emotional acceptance. In cases of stillbirth, rituals such as seeing the baby, holding it, spending time with it and having a funeral can help parents to accept the reality of what has happened.

➤ The second task is the painful process of working through the grief once the reality has been accepted. This can be a deeply agonising process, and some parents may seek to avoid the pain by making rapid changes in their lives (e.g. by moving home).

➤ Thirdly, it is necessary to adjust to life without the baby or pregnancy, which may mean that significant changes have to be made to daily routines and activities.

➤ The final task is to remember the pregnancy and the baby, but to move on with life by investing emotional energy in ongoing relationships with family and friends. This is far from suggesting that the loss is forgotten – indeed it is increasingly acknowledged that parents do not wish to forget their lost baby, but find comfort in maintaining memories of them.[8]

In reality, parents will move backwards and forwards through these phases, rather than progressing through them in a linear manner.

For many couples, deep longing for a baby and the desperate need to have another baby quickly are a way of coping with their grief (i.e. getting on with the fourth task). One bereaved mother, after the stillbirth of her son 4 months previously, called me from overseas where she was living temporarily. During a lengthy telephone conversation she spoke about her feelings of complete devastation at unexpectedly losing her son, and she described how she was scouring the Internet for anything and anyone that would help her to conceive again without delay. Her emotional recovery was not helped by her physical isolation from her friends and family, and although she was desperate for me to send her herbs to promote conception, this was not what she really required, nor what I could do for her. Instead I helped her to identify local sources of support that she could access to help her through her mourning.

Cultural variations

Cross-cultural analysis of the feelings that are experienced by women supports the view that reactions to a pregnancy loss differ widely between cultural groups,[3,9] and the kind of support that women find helpful will vary across and within communities and individuals. In a study that explored the coping strategies used by African-American women following miscarriages, ectopic pregnancies, intrauterine deaths and stillbirths, it was noted that personal relationships and religious, spiritual and cultural beliefs were significant factors in helping them to cope with their loss.[11] Organisations such as SANDS advocate ensuring that healthcare providers offer culturally relevant literature in the appropriate language, and that medical staff are aware of their own assumptions about different cultural groups in their area.

OFFERING SUPPORT
'Time heals', 'life goes on' and other unhelpful realisms

For most couples who are experiencing a pregnancy loss for the first time, it is felt as an abrupt, shattering deviation from the normal biological and social process that pregnancy is expected to follow. Nothing is ever the same again. It is a life-changing event, and for ever afterwards it serves as a marker, with other experiences being seen as occurring either before or after it.[3] It is impossible for couples to regain the pre-loss sense that pregnancy is naturally equated with parenthood. It can be agonising for some to take part in events such as Christmas, Mother's Day or other people's christenings. The social isolation that can result from this may be exacerbated by a sense that no one seems to understand or find such difficulties appropriate.

As time passes after the event, friends and family can find it difficult to appreciate that women who have experienced such a loss may still be in need years later.

> Eleanor, whose daughter was stillborn at 38 weeks, 3 years prior to starting treatment with me, expressed extreme levels of anger and bitterness when recounting her friend's recent announcement of her own pregnancy. Eleanor's anger seemed to centre on her friend's obvious joy at her pregnancy and her failure to express any caution in her view of her own pregnancy being successful. Eleanor felt that her own terrible experience had been brushed aside and belittled, and this hurt her deeply. This incident not only reawakened painful memories for her, but it also provoked such a violent emotional reaction that she was unable to control or understand herself. We agreed that she would return to counselling together with acupuncture treatment, and the combined intervention soon helped her to regain emotional equilibrium.

Women often report that the anniversary of the loss, and the date on which the baby was to be born, bring up painful memories for years after the event. Long after biomedicine has played its part, complementary medicine offers support. I have several patients who mark these dates with their own personal rituals, and seek treatment around that time to help them to cope with the emotional challenges that they pose.

Supportive work

Some of the women whom I see are seeking help several months or years after experiencing the devastation of pregnancy loss. I see others throughout their fertility journey over what can be a lengthy period, which may involve helping them through the acute intensity of grief in the immediate aftermath of a loss. In all cases it is important that I distinguish between normal and pathological grief and, where appropriate, help these women to obtain the specialist help that they may need. Pathological grief (also referred to as 'complicated' grief) is associated with the following factors, which may lead to some women being more susceptible to it:

➤ low level of social support
➤ lack of support from partner, or perceived lack of such support
➤ lower level of educational achievement
➤ previous mental health problems

➤ previous bereavements
➤ domestic violence
➤ delays in conceiving again
➤ occurrence of further adverse events.

All of those involved in caring for women who have experienced or are experiencing pregnancy loss might find that they are one of only a few people a woman may talk to. In some cases they may be the only person with whom she finds it possible to share her feelings. This is most likely to involve those who have longer-term contact with women (e.g. in primary care or, as in my case, complementary medicine). Although some women (and their partners) may need or want the specialist support of professional counselling, others simply wish to talk with and be listened to by someone supportive. When offering support to women, it is useful to listen to them and to respond to their actual needs by learning about and using helpful and comforting responses and behaviours (*see* Box 5.1).

BOX 5.1: Communication skills to facilitate supportive care

- Listen and maintain a non-judgemental attitude.
- Acknowledge the loss and offer genuine sympathy.
- Avoid making assumptions, and instead encourage expression of feelings.
- Acknowledge the feelings that are being expressed, and respond with empathy.
- Make references to the baby, and use the baby's name if the parents named him or her.
- Encourage the parents to talk to each other and to share their feelings.
- Avoid offering advice (unless this is requested) and ungrounded reassurances.

Women often welcome information about other sources of support, and offering contact details for national or local groups such as SANDS and the Miscarriage Association, or the Twins and Multiple Births Association (TAMBA), can be a useful practical support.

Although my clinical work is woman-centred, pregnancy loss affects couples, and occasionally while working with a woman after such a loss it becomes clear that her partner is in need of more support than they are receiving, although this may not yet have been recognised:

> Sasha, mother of a 4-year-old daughter, lost her second daughter as a result of a lethal abnormality at 33 weeks' gestation, when she was aged 43 years. She came to see me a year later for help with her menstrual cycle, which had not returned to normal since the pregnancy. Although Sasha felt that she had recovered emotionally and had accepted that she did not want to risk another pregnancy even if she were able to conceive again, her husband was struggling to cope, and had become overly protective towards their daughter and highly anxious about her well-being. This was affecting his work and his relationship with Sasha, their family and friends. Following my guidance, he eventually sought help from a counsellor.

REFERENCES

1 Moulder C. *Miscarriage: women's experiences and needs.* London: Routledge; 2001.
2 Raphael-Leff J. *Pregnancy: the inside story.* London: Karnac; 2001.
3 Cecil R, ed. *The Anthropology of Pregnancy Loss.* Oxford: Berg; 1996.
4 De Frain J, Millpaugh E, Xie X. The psychosocial effects of miscarriage: implications for health professionals. *Families, Systems and Health* 1996; **14:** 331–47.
5 Craig M, Tata P, Regan L. Psychiatric morbidity among patients with recurrent miscarriage. *Journal of Psychosomatic Obstetrics and Gynecology* 2002; **23:** 157–64.
6 Swanson KM, Karmali ZA, Powell SH. Miscarriage effects on couples' interpersonal and sexual relationships during the first year after loss: women's perceptions. *Psychosomatic Medicine* 2003; **65:** 902–10.
7 Laurino MY, Bennett RL, Saraiya DS *et al.* Genetic evaluation and counseling of couples with recurrent miscarriage: recommendations of the National Society of Genetic Counselors. *Journal of Genetic Counselling* 2005; **14:** 165–81.
8 Schott J, Henley A, Kohner N. *Pregnancy Loss and the Death of a Baby: guidelines for professionals.* 3rd edn. London: Sands; 2007.
9 Shaefer J. *Cross Cultural Expressions of Grief and Loss II: When an infant dies (Volume 2).* NFIMR Bulletin. Washington, DC: American College of Obstetricians and Gynecologists; 2003.
10 Worden WJ. *Grief Counseling and Grief Therapy: a handbook for the mental health professional.* 3rd edn. New York: Springer Publishing Company; 2001.
11 Van P, Meleis A. Coping with grief after involuntary pregnancy loss: perspectives of African American women. *Journal of Obstetric, Gynecologic and Neonatal Nursing* 2003; **32:** 28–39.

FURTHER READING

- Mitchell A, Cormack M. *The Therapeutic Relationship in Complementary Health Care.* Edinburgh: Churchill Livingstone; 1998.
- Watkins A. *Mind–Body Medicine: a clinician's guide to psychoneuroimmunology.* New York: Churchill Livingstone; 1997.

CHAPTER 6

Preparing for the next pregnancy

INTRODUCTION

Following a pregnancy loss, one question that is often asked is when is the right time for a couple to start trying to conceive again. In a few cases there will be medical reasons upon which to base an answer, but in most cases the response will be based on rather nebulous ideas and given in answer to a question, rather than because it is valid advice.[1] Recent research suggests that in the majority of cases there is no benefit to be gained by couples delaying pregnancy following miscarriage.[2] For some women there is no chance of another pregnancy, and they are left to cope with the double grief of losing a baby and the loss of their fertility. It is known that men and women respond differently to miscarriage, and there can be a discrepancy between when each partner feels ready to try again. In an analysis of responses from 185 women, Swanson *et al.*[3] reported that 1 year post-miscarriage, a third of women in the study described feeling more distance and less love and desire in their relationship, and regarded sexual intercourse as a functional necessity, a reminder of the loss and a source of tension.

PRECONCEPTION PREPARATION
Are tests or investigations needed?

If the parents have not seen their GP following a miscarriage – and a surprising number feel that it is not worth bothering their doctors with this – I tend to advise they do consult them to discuss their own situation and talk through any issues that may determine on a medical level when is the right time for them to try again. It may be that tests should be undertaken or referral to a specialist is needed, and a GP is best placed to manage this. There is an overwhelming need for many women to know why they miscarried or why their baby died, and what the implications are for their future pregnancies. Often the answers to these questions are not available (*see* Chapter 2), but being given the opportunity to discuss their concerns with relevant professionals is important for these women.

Preparing to try again

The time spent either waiting to feel ready to try again or for conception to occur can be difficult and fraught with mixed emotions. If the couple are actively trying to conceive, each month can be a rollercoaster of hope, optimism, anxiety and despair when the woman's period arrives. By taking an active role in her health and, even better, being joined in this by her partner, a woman can make this time seem less negative and more under her control.

Adopting a healthy diet and relationship with food

There are numerous ideas and theories about what constitutes an ideal preconception diet, and for some women this will be an area in which they want to become proactively involved, and they will benefit from this positive engagement. However, for some of the women whom I see, an obsession with what they (and their partner) should or should not be eating can lead to problems with enjoying food. It can also create feelings of failure if they 'slip' off their ideal diet, and can contribute to negative feelings about their ability to have a healthy pregnancy. Following a pregnancy loss, women's confidence can be extremely low, and I find that introducing them to ideas that focus on the enjoyment of eating in an uncomplicated and accessible way can help them to regain a sense of control over their situation.

According to traditional Chinese medicine (TCM) and dietary therapy that is based on this, health is a state of balance, which our food choices should help to create. Although some of the ideas may diverge from certain popular food fads which come in and out of fashion, they are in line with practices that have been in place for several millennia, and which have therefore stood the test of time (*see* Boxes 6.1 and 6.2). This approach also ensures that the woman obtains all of the nutrients that are generally considered to be essential for a healthy pregnancy. Using this guide as the starting point for more individualised advice, most of the women whom I see enjoy working with these ideas.

BOX 6.1: Healthy eating using traditional Chinese dietary therapy principles

Wholegrains, wholefoods and natural flavourings

- Put a strong emphasis on eating wholegrains (organic where possible), and incorporate variety. Try grains such as millet, wholewheat, oatmeal, quinoa and buckwheat. Cooking with different grains does require a little experimentation, but it can be an enriching process and enliven our interest in food.
- Strictly minimise the intake of processed foods, and eliminate ready-prepared meals from the diet. These are often high in salt, sugar and artificial chemicals.
- Use natural flavourings and sweeteners, such as honey, molasses, maple syrup, herbs and spices, rather than artificial flavourings, sweeteners, processed sugar and salt.

Fruit and vegetables

- Increase the intake of green, leafy vegetables, especially broccoli, spinach, watercress, sprouts, kale and cabbage, all of which are good sources of iron, folic acid, calcium and other essential vitamins and minerals.
- Eat a wide variety of seasonal and organic fruit and vegetables, ensuring that the five daily portions that are recommended are the minimum, while aiming for a higher intake.

Protein sources

- Eat plenty of lentils, chickpeas, kidney beans, aduki beans and other pulses.
- Obtain adequate supplies of protein from other good sources, such as organic chicken and eggs, fish, and small amounts of good-quality red meat.
- Unsalted seeds and nuts, such as almonds, macadamias, walnuts, pumpkin seeds and sunflower seeds are good sources of protein, calcium and essential fatty acids, and provide healthy snacks.

Fats
- Beneficial fats are important and should not be eliminated from our daily diet. Good choices include olive oil, dark poultry meat, nuts and avocado.

Fluids
- Strictly minimise the intake of caffeine. Instead, experiment with herbal teas. These can be an acquired taste, so persevere with them.
- Drink 2 litres of water a day (or a mixture of herbal tea and water). Start the day with a large glass of water (at room temperature) to rehydrate the body.
- Avoid fizzy drinks, and opt instead for small amounts of fruit juice or cordials.
- Limit the intake of alcohol, or give it up completely.

BOX 6.2: Healthy habits

- Follow regular eating patterns, and do not skip meals.
- Always eat breakfast, which is the most important meal in Chinese dietary therapy. It does not have to be a huge meal, but it does need to be nutritious.
- Avoid eating late at night, when it is more difficult to digest food.
- Eat according to what is in season.
- Make time to eat, and eat slowly and with enjoyment.
- Avoid overeating. Eating slowly allows time for the brain to register satiety.
- Whenever possible make lunch the main meal of the day.
- Eat meals. This sounds obvious, but people often snack or 'graze' rather than plan, prepare and cook their meals.
- Be sociable whenever possible and eat with others.
- Avoid eating when emotionally upset, tired or stressed. Take a few minutes to calm the mind before eating.

In addition, prior to conception and for the first 12 weeks of pregnancy a folic acid supplement should be taken, and women should be encouraged to maintain their BMI within the normal healthy range. Being overweight or underweight will both make it more difficult to conceive and put the pregnancy at risk. For example, overweight and obese women have higher risks of preterm labour, neonatal mortality and morbidity and very low birthweight babies,[4] and those with a BMI below $18.5\,kg/m^2$ have a higher risk of stillbirth and early miscarriage.[4,5]

Avoid known risk factors

Up to 30% of pregnant women smoke during their pregnancy,[6] and as smoking is one of the unquestionable risk factors for miscarriage, ectopic pregnancy, preterm delivery, fetal growth retardation and stillbirth,[7] it is essential that women stop smoking and using any recreational drugs when trying to conceive. It is not uncommon for women to resume smoking to relieve the stress of miscarriage, and then find it very hard to stop when they are ready to try to conceive again. Only 25% of pregnant smokers stop for even part of their pregnancy.[6] However, it is not only the physical act of smoking that presents problems to the pregnancy. Passive smoking is also known to be harmful to the fetus. Furthermore, if a woman's male partner is smoking, this reduces the likelihood of conception whether through natural means or assisted reproductive technologies.[8]

When working with women in this area, it is important to acknowledge

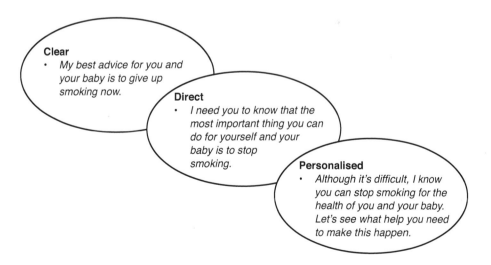

FIGURE 6.1: Use clear, direct, personalised language to encourage smoking cessation.[9]

the difficulty of quitting, and to emphasise the benefits of stopping smoking in a direct way (*see* Figure 6.1) and help women to access whatever help they need (*see* Box 6.3). Practitioners need to be mindful of how complex smoking-related issues can be and how complicated some women's lives are, provide appropriate support and remain non-judgemental.

BOX 6.3: Helping women to stop smoking

Get advice from your GP on:
- Joining a stop-smoking clinic or stop-smoking group
- Using nicotine replacement products

Plan to stop smoking by:
- Keeping a diary for 3 days noting when you smoke, how you feel at the time, and what you are doing when you have a cigarette. This will help you to see 'triggers' for smoking and help you to plan how to deal with them
- Setting a date by which you will stop smoking. This will help you to mentally prepare for it
- Telling friends and family that you are stopping, so that they can support you
- Before quitting, cleaning the car, house and furnishings, and having your teeth professionally cleaned. It will then be less appealing to contaminate them with cigarette smoke and nicotine stains

Once you decide to get started on your programme:
- Change your routines. Use the diary to show when you normally have your cigarettes. For example, if you always have a cigarette after a meal, clean your teeth instead
- Remember that the cravings will pass, and will get less and less, but think about what you will do to help them pass, such as breathing deeply, practising visualisation exercises or going out for a walk
- Find a healthy alternative to use when cravings strike. For example, prepare some carrot sticks and keep them handy, or chew gum, or make a telephone call to a supportive friend
- Be positive and keep reminding yourself why you want to stop smoking and the health risks of not doing so
- Keep busy, and take up an activity that makes it hard to smoke, such as swimming

---

The most effective way of stopping smoking at present appears to be a combination of behavioural support and nicotine replacement therapy (NRT). However, it is difficult for health professionals to provide clear unequivocal guidance to pregnant women on the safety of using NRT, as it has yet to be studied thoroughly during pregnancy. What evidence there is remains inconclusive, although there is expert consensus that NRT is safer than smoking in pregnancy so long as the levels of nicotine remain lower than those obtained by smoking.[6] It may be worth considering alternative methods of encouraging smoking cessation, such as hypnosis or acupuncture, and there are practitioners who are experts in this field. Whatever their stage of pregnancy, it is always worthwhile for pregnant women to reduce their cigarette consumption, and although total cessation is the aim, any reduction is better than none.

Managing stress
During the period before a woman attempts to conceive again, it is helpful if she can be encouraged to find practical ways to reduce the stressful demands on her and learn techniques for managing stress and anxiety. This is especially valuable prior to conception because the post-loss pregnancy is normally fraught with anxiety, and it can be a long and trying time before the woman feels safe in her pregnancy. Therefore the more confident she can feel about her stress management strategies, the more effectively these will see her through the pregnancy. Women may worry that if they are unable to control their anxiety or fears, this will harm either their ability to conceive again, or the pregnancy should it occur. There is some evidence that these fears have validity. A recent study[4] found that women who reported feeling 'happy', 'relaxed' or 'in control' during the first 12 weeks of their pregnancy had a lower incidence of first-trimester miscarriage compared with the other women in the study. Conversely, those who reported feeling stressed, anxious, depressed, out of control or overwhelmed during the same period had a much higher incidence of miscarriage. Furthermore, there was a strong trend towards a greater likelihood of miscarrying if the woman had a stressful or demanding job.

Nakamura *et al.*,[10] in a large-scale review of epidemiological studies published over the last three decades, have presented convincing evidence for biological mechanisms involving an immune–endocrine disequilibrium in response to stress and reproductive failure. Notably, the review identifies links between stress perception and pregnancy outcome. It has been shown that factors which affect how an individual responds to stress include personality traits, early life experiences and learned coping strategies.[11] Research does suggest that if individuals are helped to redefine difficult circumstances relating to their health, in this case reproductive health, in positive ways, this has benefits for psychological well-being. Positive reappraisal may involve encouraging women to focus on the positive aspects of the situation (e.g. the improvement in general health and well-being arising from lifestyle changes, or the fact that their partner is more supportive or caring than previously). Certainly research supports this positive approach in other areas of health-related difficulties, such as infertility, breast cancer and bereavement,[12] and there is no reason to doubt the validity of the approach in many areas of healthcare. Complementary and alternative medicine (CAM) offers great potential in relation to this aspect, and is covered in Chapter 7. However, there are a number of simple strategies that women can be encouraged to adopt, and which they can fit into their daily lives.

➤ Using something as simple as worry beads can have the effect of reducing physical and emotional tension, and this handy method can achieve a real sense of general relaxation.

➤ Visualisation can be taught in a structured way as part of a wide-ranging stress management approach, but it can be as simple as focusing attention on visualising a pleasant place where one is relaxed or happy, such as a summer garden, a sandy beach on holiday, or an autumn wood. The place only needs to have a positive meaning for the person who is visualising it, and this can be enough to stop them thinking about stress or anxiety-generating issues, which in turn lowers overall tension.

➤ Take regular warm baths. This will physically relax tense muscles and mentally allow the mind to still itself. Some of the women whom I see say that they do not have time to take baths, and they only have quick showers. This in itself reveals the hectic pace at which they are living, and the low priority that they are giving to relaxation for themselves.

➤ Adopt a regular exercise programme.

➤ I encourage my patients to allocate at least one hour a day entirely to themselves. This is time that they use for their own pleasure, not for rushing round the supermarket or doing the ironing (unless ironing gives them pleasure!). They do not need to fill this time with activity.

It can be spent sitting quietly in the garden doing nothing, or taking a bath. Whatever they do, it is an hour (at least) that is not crowded or even productive in the sense of achieving anything more than a sense of calm.

➤ Learn to meditate. Anyone can meditate, but many people struggle to do it at first or may be resistant to the idea, perhaps fearing that it is too peculiar or weird for them. I provide a simple set of instructions (*see* Box 6.4) to get people started, and encourage further exploration through extra reading material and resources.

I advise women to try as many of these techniques as possible regularly, and to keep a record of how they feel after each of them. This helps them to discover which of the approaches is best for them, and it inspires them to continue with the techniques over the long term.

BOX 6.4: Everyday ways to meditate in order to reduce stress

Breathe deeply

- This is one of the most important tools for reducing stress. Either lie or sit comfortably in a quiet place. Focus all your attention on your breathing. Place one hand on your chest and the other on your tummy. Close your eyes and concentrate on feeling and listening as you breathe in through your nose and out through your mouth. Breathe deeply and slowly. Feel your chest rise, and with each intake of breath take it a little deeper into your abdomen, which you should feel expand. When your attention wanders, gently return your focus to your breathing, perhaps silently saying 'In' and 'Out' as you rhythmically and slowly inhale and exhale. Do this exercise for 15 minutes at least a couple of times a day, and after a week or so this will become your normal way of breathing to calm and settle your stresses.

Scan your body

- Sit or lie comfortably, with your eyes closed, and focus on your body in careful and minute detail. Sense every muscle from the tips of your toes to the top of your head. Be aware of any tension, pain, warmth or cold, and relax any tension that you feel. Combine body scanning with breathing deeply, and imagine breathing warmth and relaxation into and out of different parts of your body.

Repeat a mantra
- A mantra is a word or phrase that is either spoken or thought repeatedly as a way of focusing the mind. It can be any phrase, sound or word that you find useful to repeat.

Meditation is a learned skill and it takes practice. It is common for our minds to wander during meditation. When this happens, slowly refocus on the object, sensation or mantra. Experiment and you will find out what works best for you and what you enjoy. The beauty of meditation is that we can adapt it to our needs at any moment. There is no right or wrong way to meditate. The most important thing is that it helps you to reduce your stress.

Exercise

Moderate exercise throughout pregnancy is beneficial, and it should be encouraged prior to conception both to help with weight management if this is a problem, and to regulate stress. Some of the women I see who have miscarried cease all physical activities when trying to conceive again. There is no evidence to support this over-cautious approach. Overall, the evidence on whether exercise in pregnancy contributes to adverse pregnancy outcomes such as preterm labour points to the benefits of moderate, supervised exercise such as swimming, light weight exercises and yoga, even in women who before they became pregnant had a sedentary lifestyle.[13] I encourage women to modify their exercise regime if necessary, or to try new forms of exercise, such as yoga, swimming or walking, but not to stop exercising completely. Yoga is probably one of the world's oldest forms of exercise, and modern research supports its use in reducing stress during pregnancy,[14] increasing the birth weight of babies, and lowering the incidence of intrauterine growth retardation and preterm labour.[15] One of the most important things that a woman can do when preparing for pregnancy is to find activities which she enjoys. Whatever she chooses, the activity should not contribute to negative thoughts or generate any anxieties within her.

Screening for and preventing infections

Given that some infections are associated with adverse pregnancy outcomes or reduced fertility, it may be appropriate to advise women on how to decrease their risk of contracting infections during pregnancy. In particular, once they are pregnant, women should be advised to avoid handling cat litter or animal faeces, to wear gloves when gardening, to practise strict hygiene and handwashing after coming into contact with the urine, saliva or nappies of young children, and to avoid eating or handling raw or under-cooked meat. Screening of both partners for sexually transmitted infections may be advisable if there are delays in conceiving, and should be seen as a positive step, as most common infections can be treated, but a high degree of sensitivity may be required with some couples. Women should ensure that they are up to date with vaccinations such as rubella.

REFERENCES

1 Moulder C. *Miscarriage: women's experiences and needs.* London: Routledge; 2001.

2 Love ER, Bhattacharya S, Smith NC *et al.* Effect of interpregnancy interval on outcomes of pregnancy after miscarriage: retrospective analysis of hospital episode statistics in Scotland. *BMJ* 2010; **341:** c3967.

3 Swanson KM, Karmali ZA, Powell SH. Miscarriage effects on couples' interpersonal and sexual relationships during the first year after loss: women's perceptions. *Psychosomatic Medicine* 2003; **65:** 902–10.

4 Maconochie N, Doyle P, Prior S *et al.* Risk factors for first trimester miscarriage – results from a UK-population-based case–control study. *British Journal of Obstetrics and Gynaecology* 2007; **114:** 170–86.

5 Confidential Enquiry into Maternal and Child Health (CEMACH). *Perinatal Mortality 2007: United Kingdom.* London: CEMACH; 2009.

6 Coleman T, Thornton J, Britton J *et al.* Protocol for the Smoking, Nicotine and Pregnancy (SNAP) trial: double-blind, placebo-randomised, controlled trial of nicotine replacement therapy in pregnancy. *BMC Health Services Research* 2007; **7:** 2.

7 Högberg L, Cnattingius S. The influence of maternal smoking habits on the risk of subsequent stillbirth: is there a causal relation? *British Journal of Obstetrics and Gynaecology* 2007; **114:** 699–704.

8 British Medical Association. *Smoking and Reproductive Life: the impact of smoking on sexual, reproductive and child health.* www.bma.org.uk/images/smoking_tcm41-21289.pdf (accessed 20 August 2010).

9 American Congress of Obstetricians and Gynecologists. *Smoking Cessation Presentation.* www.acog.org/ACOG_Sections/dist_notice.cfm?recno=4&bulletin=1804 (accessed 20 August 2010).

10 Nakamura K, Sheps S, Arck PC. Stress and reproductive failure: past notions, present insights and future directions. *Journal of Assisted Reproduction and Genetics* 2008; **25:** 47–62.

11 Hogue CJR, Hoffman S, Hatch MC. Stress and preterm delivery: a conceptual framework. *Paediatric and Perinatal Epidemiology* 2001; **15 (Suppl. 2):** 30–40.

12 Lancastle D, Boivin J. A feasibility study of a brief coping intervention (PRCI) for the waiting period before a pregnancy test during fertility treatment. *Human Reproduction* 2008; **23:** 2299–307.

13 Barakat R, Stirling JR, Lucia A. Does exercise training during pregnancy affect gestational age? A randomised controlled trial. *British Journal of Sports Medicine* 2008; **42:** 674–8.

14 Satyapriyaa M, Nagendraa HR, Nagarathnaa R *et al.* Effect of integrated yoga on stress and heart rate variability in pregnant women. *International Journal of Gynecology and Obstetrics* 2009; **104:** 218–22.

15 Narendran S, Nagarathna R, Gunasheela S *et al.* Efficacy of yoga in pregnant women with abnormal Doppler study of umbilical and uterine arteries. *Journal of the Indian Medical Association* 2005; **103:** 12–17.

FURTHER READING

- Pitchford P. *Healing with Whole Foods.* 3rd edn. Berkeley, CA: North Atlantic Books; 2002.
- Pollan M. *In Defence of Food.* London: Allen Lane; 2008.

CHAPTER 7

Complementary and alternative medicine in context

INTRODUCTION

Traditional therapies have been used throughout history to promote the health and well-being of women during pregnancy. According to the World Health Organization (WHO), 65–80% of the world's population use traditional medicine.[1] The modalities embodied by complementary and alternative medicine (CAM) are in large part based upon traditional medicine. These practices can be dismissed prematurely by some for a number of reasons. The unfamiliar language that is sometimes used to describe what is done, the 'New Age' tone of some CAM exponents, and the extravagant claims that are occasionally made, coupled with the limited scientific evidence for many therapies, can all create an unappealing impression. Alongside this there are concerns about the safety of such therapies. However, for the majority of the professionally administered therapies, when due consideration is given to the nature of the therapies and the available evidence, these concerns can be addressed. Increasing numbers of women are using CAM during pregnancy, and according to the WHO the reasons for this general increase in use of CAM include concerns about the adverse effects of pharmaceuticals, a wish for more personalised healthcare, and greater public access to health information.[2] The holistic approach to health and the encouragement of individual patient empowerment that are central to most CAM practices do have a place in prevention of and recovery from miscarriage and pregnancy loss. The growing professionalism of the more established therapies, such as hypnosis and acupuncture, ensures improved access to well-trained, competent practitioners who understand the multiple, complex issues that may be involved. This chapter explores key themes relating to CAM in this field, as well as identifying areas where it can play a significant and beneficial role for women.

DEFINING CAM

Complementary and alternative medicine encompasses a great range of treatments and activities, but at present there is no universally accepted definition of CAM. In the USA, the National Center for Complementary and Alternative Medicine (NCCAM) suggests that CAM refers to diverse medical and healthcare systems, practices and products that are not generally considered to be part of conventional or orthodox medicine.[3] Similarly, in the UK, the complementary and alternative medicine section on the NHS Evidence website describes a set of therapies, practices and approaches to healthcare that lie outside mainstream conventional medicine. In addition, the term *integrated medicine* has more recently been used to refer to those therapies that are available within an institution or practice.[4] In Australia, the National Institute of Complementary Medicine has adapted the NCCAM definition, and favours *complementary medicine (CM)* as an inclusive term to represent a range of medicines and therapies that are concerned with both the maintenance of wellness and the treatment of illness, but which are not considered to be part of core conventional medicine.

There are several ways to group the various therapies and practices, and Box 7.1 summarises the most common groups. The distinctions between categories are not rigid, and there are several potential crossovers between therapies (e.g. aromatherapy utilises aromatic essential oils as well as massage). Neither are the boundaries between CAM and conventional medicine absolute, and some CAM practices are increasingly being accepted into mainstream medicine.[2]

BOX 7.1: Broad categories for CAM practices with examples of those that are most commonly available (note that some therapies can be placed in more than one category)

Biological – natural product-based

- Aromatic essential oils
- Dietary supplements such as vitamins and minerals
- Herbs

Mind–body medicine
- Art, music and drama therapy
- Guided imagery and visualisation
- Hypnotherapy
- Meditation
- Mindfulness therapy
- Relaxation therapy

Manipulative and body-based
- Aromatherapy
- Chiropractic
- Indian head massage
- Massage
- Osteopathy
- Reflexology
- T'ai chi
- Yoga

Energy medicine
- Flower remedies
- Magnet therapy
- Reiki
- Therapeutic touch

Whole medical systems
These encompass many of the other categories, and are built upon complete systems of theory and practice
- Chinese medicine (i.e. acupuncture, herbs, dietary therapy and massage)
- Ayurvedic medicine
- Naturopathy
- Homeopathy

THE USE OF CAM IN OBSTETRICS
Prevalence of use
Historically, women have been the main users of complementary therapies, and this includes their use during pregnancy.[5] Although it is difficult to

identify accurately the number of people who are currently using CAM, there is sufficient evidence to suggest that its use has increased in the past couple of decades, both generally and within obstetrics.[2,6,7] One barrier to obtaining accurate information about the actual number of people who use CAM is the 'pervasive silence' and 'professional disinterest' that has been described in relation to its use, and reluctance of patients to discuss it with their doctors in case they meet with disapproval.[8,9]

In Germany, CAM methods such as acupuncture, homeopathy and aromatherapy are available in most obstetric departments.[10] In the USA it is recognised that one of the largest groups of CAM users consists of educated, employed women of reproductive age.[5] A 2004 report[11] on the attitudes and referral patterns of Australian midwives and obstetricians found that the majority had formally referred a patient for at least one of the complementary therapies, with over 70% of obstetricians and midwives regarding massage, acupuncture, vitamins, yoga, meditation and hypnosis as useful and safe to use during pregnancy. Worldwide surveys have consistently highlighted the popularity of the use of herbal therapy by pregnant women, often through recommendations from family and friends rather than under professional guidance.[6,12]

Although there is a lack of quantifying data specifically relating to CAM use by women who have experienced pregnancy loss, surveys have found higher rates of use among infertility patients than in the general population.[13] Although it cannot be said for certain that the same pattern would be found in women who have lost pregnancies, this is not an unreasonable assumption, as the needs and motivations of women in both situations are often very similar.

Safety

Although the safety of many CAM therapies has not been studied in widespread clinical trials, most of these therapies have a good safety record. Several of them have been used for hundreds or even thousands of years with little if any evidence of harm, and furthermore many CAM therapies seem to have little potential for causing harm.[14] For most therapies there is a strong documented history of indications for use, along with relevant cautions or contraindications for use in certain circumstances, including pregnancy. These are fully understood by trained professional practitioners who have confidence in their own knowledge and limitations. As a practitioner of one the oldest extant medical systems, Chinese medicine, my professional standpoint is that what I and my colleagues offer women is a therapy that has a well-documented historical lineage from which practitioners draw their knowledge. As well as this empirically robust and abundant scholarly source, there are increasing numbers of high-quality studies which demonstrate that professionally administered acupuncture during pregnancy is safe and effective, with very few safety concerns. Furthermore, studies show that it is not associated with adverse outcomes.[15-17] A loose parallel in mainstream reproductive medicine where there is a low level of scientifically sound evidence about the use of a therapy can be seen with the current use of progesterone supplementation in early pregnancy following IVF – a practice for which there is limited evidence of benefit, but decades of use showing no serious side-effects.[18,19]

Barriers that prevent wider use of CAM
Although scientific explanations of how many CAM therapies work are lacking, this should not prevent the considered use of appropriate therapies by those who seek to improve their physical and emotional health and the likelihood of a successful pregnancy. In an interesting paper examining the reasons why male cancer patients choose to use CAM, it was reported that some men, notably from a scientific background, identified limitations in the scientific evidence-based approach to conventional treatments, and did not equate lack of scientific evidence for CAM with lack of effectiveness.[8] Some practices face prejudice and misunderstanding, as has been the case until recent years with hypnotherapy, a therapy that is steadily gaining a valuable place in obstetric care, despite many years of suspicion about and hostility towards its use.[20] One reason why medical professionals and scientists are sometimes put off or at the very least sceptical about therapies such as homeopathy or acupuncture is that even if it is accepted that they may be safe and effective in some cases, they work in ways that science cannot yet explain. In a society where the scientific method is dominant, it is understandable that this poses problems. However, many allopathic approaches are not evidence-based, some remain highly controversial, yet many produce positive outcomes. The ability of patients to carefully and deliberately integrate CAM and medical approaches to their health should not be underestimated. It is far from haphazard or driven by desperation, as it has occasionally been depicted in the conventional medical literature.[9]

The long history and enduring use of many therapies have been cited by patients as indicators of their effectiveness and benefit.[8] This should not be lightly dismissed when the traditional 'paternalistic' nature of the doctor–patient relationship is shifting to one in which the patient is encouraged to take greater responsibility for their health and treatment choices.[8] Viewed in this context, traditional therapies have a place so long as they are used under the guidance of well-trained specialist practitioners who are familiar with all of the issues involved. Certain therapies may bring much benefit and no harm to women, and there are many good reasons for exploring them.

The role of the CAM practitioner

Despite the considerable clinical experience and research efforts of medical professionals working in the field, mainstream conventional medicine does not yet have all the answers to help women who have experienced pregnancy loss. Doctors and healthcare professionals are working within the limitations of the knowledge that is currently available, and great gaps in knowledge still exist. In the absence of an identifiable and treatable reason for miscarriage, it is important that women keep trying to conceive for as long as they feel able to and, more importantly, wish to do so, as for the majority there will eventually be a successful pregnancy.[19] However, a sense of optimism is very hard to sustain in the face of one loss after another, and it is here that CAM therapies can offer much support on the journey, both physically and emotionally. The concept of personal and social resilience in people who have experienced trauma and loss has been defined as the ability to maintain stable, healthy levels of psychological and physical functioning. In a small study, researchers identified women who received acupuncture (in this particular study alongside infertility treatment) describing pathways to resilience.[21] The study participants perceived many benefits of acupuncture, including the way that it addressed aspects of their emotions that were neglected in conventional medicine. They described a sense of emotional stability, an improved sense of coping, self-confidence, cognitive clarity and processing of negative feelings that changed to more positive and optimistic attitudes through the holistic caring approach of the practitioner.[21]

Women vary greatly in how much medical help they seek following miscarriage, and some are more comfortable with CAM practitioners, who often spend more time with their patients than those working in mainstream healthcare. The limited amount of time that conventional practitioners can spend with their patients has been identified as one of the main reasons why many patients are turning to CAM.[22] From a holistic perspective, CAM treatment effects are thought to arise in part from sources related to the therapeutic relationship between patient and practitioner.[23,24] Seeking help from a therapist can be very helpful in itself, and the process of doing something for herself and being listened to can help a woman to gain a sense of control over the situation and her health. The emphasis that most CAM practices place on the subjective experience of the patient, with a focus on the whole patient and the context of their family, work and overall lifestyle,[22] makes CAM an attractive choice for many women who are recovering from a lost pregnancy.

Women can sometimes feel that doctors are being evasive or unhelpful – for example, when they do not recommend starting investigations or treatment,[25] especially if the reasons for this are poorly communicated. When a trusted practitioner provides reassurance that what is being suggested is in the woman's best interests and is appropriate, this can be perceived by the woman as very supportive. On the other hand, a well-informed and knowledgeable therapist may sometimes make suggestions for seeking further help or referral if the patient has not seen their GP or has not been offered help that may be available. As discussed elsewhere, medical staff are not always as sensitive and understanding as they might be in cases of early miscarriage, and this can cause profound distress to the women concerned, who may actively seek the support and advice of a CAM practitioner:

> Rowena, aged 41 years, had experienced an early miscarriage some years before seeing me, and it had been several years before she subsequently conceived, 4 months after starting acupuncture treatment. She experienced bleeding at 8 weeks and went straight to her GP practice in a state of high anxiety, where the practice nurse on duty informed her that the risks of miscarriage were very high at her age, and she should not have been surprised to find herself in this situation. Rowena was told to go away and 'expect the worst.' She phoned me in a distraught state, asking for advice, and I suggested that she should contact her local Early Pregnancy Unit (EPU) immediately, as they would be able to assess the situation. At the unit she was sensitively treated and reassured that although it was a threatened miscarriage, it was not inevitable that she would miscarry. She eventually went on to deliver a healthy baby girl.

This case highlights the fact that although the practice nurse was statistically correct, and the likelihood of miscarriage was indeed high, this was not a helpful response and it served only to compound the patient's distress. Being aware of the role of the Early Pregnancy Unit and referring this woman on would have been more appropriate, as would a compassionate and thoughtful attitude.

Reducing stress and anxiety

Over the past couple of decades, numerous studies have provided convincing evidence that negative maternal emotional states during pregnancy are associated with adverse pregnancy outcomes. The association between high levels of maternal anxiety and stress and preterm delivery and low birth weight for gestational age are the most replicated findings.[26] There are suggestions from some studies that women perceive negative events as more distressing when they occur during the first trimester as compared with the last trimester of pregnancy.[27] Therefore it is important that treatments which aim to reduce the impact of emotional stress are implemented from the earliest stages of pregnancy. Abnormal blood flow in the uterine arteries, which is linked to adverse pregnancy outcomes such as intrauterine growth restriction and pre-eclampsia, has been found in several studies involving highly anxious women, and may account for some cases of poor obstetric outcome.[26] However, it is entirely possible that in some cases the mother may be aware of existing pregnancy complications, which in turn leads to anxiety. In other words, anxiety may not always be an independent risk factor. Nevertheless, identifying women with high levels of anxiety may help to detect those at risk of preterm labour, and measures can then be sought to help to relieve the anxiety and lower the risk. Major psychological changes occur in the last weeks of pregnancy, specifically mood disturbances, including a significant rise in the levels of anger, confusion and tension from 28–38 weeks.[27]

Many CAM therapies have a good track record for alleviating anxiety and depression and reducing stress in the general and pregnant population, with some supporting evidence from clinical trials and systematic reviews.[4,28] In a recent trial of pregnant women who were diagnosed with depression, those who received twice-weekly massage therapy showed a greater decrease in depression and anxiety compared with the control group. They also showed a reduction in depression during the postpartum period, and their babies were less likely to be born prematurely or with low birth weight.[29] Several studies have shown that acupuncture induces a state of relaxation and improves mild to moderate emotional complaints during pregnancy.[30,31] In a case series, Johnson[32] reported that a notable calming effect was achieved with acupuncture during IVF treatment, and suggested an association with the improvement in pregnancy rate in the group.

Tender loving care

In 1984, researchers first highlighted the importance of reassurance and what was termed 'tender loving care' for women who were experiencing recurrent miscarriage.[33] Subsequent work has repeatedly shown that in cases of recurrent miscarriage with no identified cause, the provision of regular scans and reassurance that the pregnancy was progressing in the first trimester significantly improved the likelihood of successful pregnancy. In one of the largest studies a successful pregnancy was achieved in 75% of cases.[34] These incredibly positive findings highlight the enormous value of women being cared for by professionals who respect and listen to them, allow them to express their feelings or concerns, and provide appropriate reassurances and care. If a woman is anxious about how her pregnancy is progressing, I always advise a visit to her midwife or EPU, as she will then obtain accurate information, hopefully be reassured that all is well and not be left with her anxious thoughts lying unaddressed. Conventional healthcare providers often struggle to understand the unique circumstances presented by individual women,[35] and on occasion fail to demonstrate a caring and empathic attitude at a time when this might make the difference between a successful pregnancy and one that fails. The very nature of many CAM practices can overcome some of the problems here, as the holistic theoretical models that are used often involve exploration of the emotional realm and connections between the soma and the psyche. Voicing their concerns can greatly help women to progress through their pregnancy in a calmer emotional state.

Identifying coping resources and sources of support

Poor personal coping resources may increase the risk of adverse pregnancy outcomes. High self-esteem and a perception of control over one's life are recognised as coping resources that buffer the effects of stress,[36] but pregnancy loss can have a devastating effect on a woman's self-esteem and confidence. A common theme that emerges in my clinical practice is that healthcare professionals often do not understand or at least do not appear to understand the powerful feelings that miscarriage engenders in women, especially when the loss occurs early and medically the event is almost a 'non-event.' Therefore, although the physical experience of miscarriage may have occurred weeks or even months previously, exploring the emotional reactions to that experience within the therapeutic encounter of CAM practice can have very positive effects for many women, enabling them to make personal sense of their loss and to move on. Not infrequently I find that my patients share thoughts and memories with me that they have not shared with anyone else. Although it cannot be claimed that the experiences described to me are representative of other women visiting CAM practitioners, neither is there any reason to think that they are atypical. In a small exploratory study of women's experiences of receiving acupuncture alongside IVF treatment, the study participants described experiencing a nurturing peaceful physical space while they underwent acupuncture, in which they found emotional space to express their feelings. All of them described the sense of social support that they felt through the therapeutic encounter and the compassionate care that they received.[21] The availability of emotionally supportive individuals, whether they are professionals, friends or family, can help to alleviate the feelings of failure, anger, shame, guilt, longing, depression and insecurity that are so commonly experienced following a loss – feelings that can persist well into a woman's subsequent pregnancy. The effects of social support on maternal emotional health and pregnancy outcome are considerable, and many studies have demonstrated adverse outcomes in women with low levels of social support.[37] In the weeks and months following a loss, CAM practitioners can be a unique source of support, as well as encouraging women to access other sources of help, such as local or national support groups, or improving her social integration, all of which will help to prepare her for a subsequent pregnancy, and help her through it when it occurs.

Supporting empowerment
The idea and popularity of 'patient empowerment' have arisen in recent years within the context of greater individual health responsibility, the development of the health consumer and moves to involve patients in treatment decision making. Most CAM practices facilitate the active engagement of individuals in their health. Within acupuncture practice, a pattern

of individualised patient-centred care based on a therapeutic partnership and close involvement of patients in their treatment has been identified.[31] Another element of acupuncture practice that empowers women is the use of explanatory models from Chinese medicine theory, which aid the development of their understanding of their condition. The use of simple, everyday language by CAM practitioners to explain their models of health and understanding of disease can facilitate a more comfortable fit between the patient's view and that of their practitioner.[22] This approach makes it easier to motivate lifestyle changes that reinforce the potential for health and well-being, in contrast to the technical and sometimes bewildering language that is used in conventional medicine.

THE NEXT PREGNANCY
Preconception care

In medicine, there is little agreement on how long after a miscarriage a couple should wait before trying to conceive again, with some clinicians advising delaying for several months and others seeing little justification for this. Recent research concurs with the latter view, and in the absence of medical problems such as infection, it seems unnecessary to recommend that women delay conception.[38] Whenever a couple decides to try for another pregnancy following a loss, they should be encouraged to prepare well both physically and emotionally, and to find practical ways of reducing their stress and anxiety. Many CAM therapies focus strongly on positive lifestyle choices and healthy practices, and adopting such measures can greatly help couples to gain a perception of control over their situation. If a woman is smoking, several CAM therapies have a good track record in smoking cessation programmes and should be considered. The interventions that are most commonly reported to be of benefit are hypnotherapy, relaxation, acupuncture, meditation, yoga and massage.[39]

Key areas about which CAM practitioners are often highly knowledgeable and best placed to offer guidance (depending on the particular therapeutic discipline) include the following:

➤ adopting optimal healthy eating habits in order to achieve optimum pre-conception nutritional status and weight

➤ giving advice on taking appropriate dietary supplements

➤ help with supporting both partners, not just the mother, to stop smoking

➤ encouraging and assisting both partners to keep alcohol intake within the recommended limits for conception and pregnancy

➤ encouraging and teaching specific relaxation techniques to reduce anxiety

➤ offering time and the opportunity for the parents to discuss their feelings, and if necessary helping them to access specialist counselling or psychotherapeutic help.

There is some evidence that those who take longer to conceive following a miscarriage have more difficulties in coping, and experience increased levels of despair.[40] Some CAM therapies have a long tradition of promoting natural conception, and if delays in conceiving are compounding the distress, they may be worth considering for this aspect alone.

During the pregnancy

Although every pregnancy is unique, and it is never possible to predict how a couple will feel during another pregnancy, overwhelming anxiety and worry are very typical. Mothers are often hypervigilant and seek constant reassurance that all is well with the pregnancy. This has been identified by researchers as a common coping mechanism for some women,[41] which healthcare providers need to recognise. In a thorough literature review of parental experiences during post-loss pregnancies, Hill *et al.*[42] have highlighted the importance to women of healthcare providers acknowledging and validating their loss. Furthermore, women wish to see their concerns being taken seriously during any subsequent pregnancy. Encouraging women to talk about their emotions and concerns throughout the pregnancy is vital, and the therapeutic space provided by many CAM practices lends itself well to this area of care. Particular dates and stages can be distressing for parents – for example, the anniversary of the loss or the day that the lost baby would have been due – and arranging treatment sessions to coincide with these dates can be highly beneficial.

Preterm labour risk and multiple pregnancy

If there is a previous history of stillbirth, preterm labour or complications in a previous pregnancy, or it is a multiple pregnancy, women will normally be seen in special consultant-led clinics to ensure close monitoring and care. Although this specialist approach provides welcome reassurance for most couples, it can have some disadvantages, as contact with other parents with high-risk pregnancies can heighten fears and worries.[43] The non-medicalised and understanding nature of most CAM practices can provide a useful supplement to the support provided by medical staff, thus ensuring that parents feel they have been attended to adequately.

In view of the known risk factors for preterm labour, and the risks associated with multiple pregnancies, identifying these and educating and supporting women with regard to making any necessary changes to their lifestyle should be part of routine medical care. The unique role of the CAM practitioner can supplement, rather than replace, the help that is provided through conventional care. The following areas can be discussed and addressed as appropriate.

➤ Encourage early and regular antenatal care, as well as additional scans or antenatal appointments if the couple requires extra reassurance about the progress of their pregnancy.

➤ Evaluate home and work stress, and advise on appropriate modifications to lifestyle.

➤ Assess the woman's support systems and coping mechanisms, and discourage behaviours that put her under additional pressure, such as working excessively long hours or delaying taking maternity leave.

➤ Encourage the woman to rest during the day, especially as the pregnancy progresses, to avoid putting undue pressure on the cervix.

➤ Provide guidance on suitable forms of exercise to decrease fatigue and stress, such as pregnancy yoga under the guidance of a specialist teacher.

➤ Teach and encourage the use of relaxation techniques to reduce the effects of stress (*see* Chapter 6).

Women can feel much more resourceful, physically healthy and more in control during their subsequent pregnancies when using many CAM practices.

REFERENCES

1 World Health Organization. *Factsheet No.134: Traditional Medicine.* www.who.int/ mediacentre/factsheets/fs134/en/ print.html (accessed 11 January 2010).

2 Falkenberg T. Session 63: Paramedical Debate Session 'Alternative Medicine, Patients

Feeling in Control?' O-251 From alternative medicine towards integrative care – health care providers and patients need for control? *Human Reproduction* 2010; **25 (Suppl. 1):** i98–9.

3 http://nccam.nih.gov/health/whatiscam/#types

4 NHS Evidence – Complementary and Alternative Medicine. *2008 Annual Evidence Update on CAM in Depression: massage, aromatherapy and reflexology.* www.library.nhs.uk//cam/ViewResource.aspx?resID=295216 (accessed 29 September 2010).

5 Furlow ML, Patel DA, Sen A *et al.* Physician and patient attitudes towards complementary and alternative medicine in obstetrics and gynecology. *BMC Complementary and Alternative Medicine* 2008; **8:** 35.

6 Forster DA, Denning A, Wills G *et al.* Herbal medicine use during pregnancy in a group of Australian women. *BMC Pregnancy and Childbirth* 2006; **6:** 21.

7 Petrie KA, Peck MR. Alternative medicine in maternity care. *Primary Care* 2000; **27:** 117–36.

8 Evans M, Shaw A, Thompson EA *et al.* Decisions to use complementary and alternative medicine (CAM) by male cancer patients: information-seeking roles and types of evidence used. *BMC Complementary and Alternative Medicine* 2007; **7:** 25.

9 Adler SR. Relationships among older patients, CAM practitioners, and physicians: the advantages of qualitative inquiry. *Alternative Therapies in Health and Medicine* 2003; **9:** 104–10.

10 Münstedt K, Brenken A, Kalder M. Clinical indications and perceived effectiveness of complementary and alternative medicine in departments of obstetrics in Germany: a questionnaire study. *European Journal of Obstetrics, Gynecology and Reproductive Biology* 2009; **146:** 50–54.

11 Gaffney L, Smith CA. Use of complementary therapies in pregnancy: the perceptions of obstetricians and midwives in South Australia. *Australian and New Zealand Journal of Obstetrics and Gynaecology* 2004; **44:** 24–9.

12 Holst L, Wright D, Haavik S *et al.* The use and the user of herbal remedies during pregnancy. *Journal of Alternative and Complementary Medicine* 2009; **15:** 787–92.

13 Coulson C, Jenkins J. Complementary and alternative medicine utilisation in NHS and private clinic settings: a United Kingdom survey of 400 infertility patients. *Journal of Experimental and Clinical Assisted Reproduction* 2005; **2:** 5.

14 Porter RS, Kaplan JL, eds. *The Merck Manual for Healthcare Professionals.* Whitehouse Station, NJ: Merck Sharp & Dohme Corp; 2010. www.merck.com/mmpe/sec22/ch330/ch330a.html (accessed 23 September 2010).

15 Smith C, Dahlen H. Caring for the pregnant woman and her baby in a changing maternity service environment: the role of acupuncture. *Acupuncture in Medicine* 2009; **27:** 123–5.

16 Smith CA, Cochrane S. Does acupuncture have a place as an adjunct treatment during pregnancy? A review of randomized controlled trials and systematic reviews. *Birth* 2009; **36**: 246–53.

17 Smith C, Crowther C, Beilby J. Pregnancy outcome following women's participation in a randomised controlled trial of acupuncture to treat nausea and vomiting in early pregnancy. *Complementary Therapies in Medicine* 2002; **10**: 78–83.

18 Oates-Whitehead RM, Haas DM, Carrrier JA. Progestogen for preventing miscarriage. *Cochrane Database of Systematic Reviews* 2003; **4**: CD003511.

19 Cohen J. *Coming to Term*. New Brunswick, NJ: Rutgers University Press; 2007.

20 Cyna AM, Andrew MI, Robinson JS. Hypnosis antenatal training for childbirth (HATCh): a randomised controlled trial. *BMC Pregnancy and Childbirth*. 2006; **6**: 5.

21 De Lacey S, Smith CA, Paterson C. Building resilience: a preliminary exploration of women's perceptions of the use of acupuncture as an adjunct to *in vitro* fertilisation. *BMC Complementary and Alternative Medicine* 2009; **9**: 50.

22 House of Lords Select Committee on Science and Technology. *Session 1999–2000, Sixth Report. Complementary and Alternative Medicine. HL Paper 123*. London: The Stationery Office; 2000. www.publications.parliament.uk/pa/ld199900/ldselect/ldsctech/123/12302.htm (accessed 2 September 2010).

23 Bann CM, Sirois FM, Walsh EG. Provider support in complementary and alternative medicine: exploring the role of patient empowerment. *Journal of Alternative and Complementary Medicine* 2010; **16**: 745–52.

24 Paterson C, Britten N. Acupuncture as a complex intervention: a holistic model. *Journal of Alternative and Complementary Medicine* 2004; **10**: 791–801.

25 Moulder C. *Miscarriage: women's experiences and needs*. London: Routledge; 2001.

26 Van den Bergh BRH, Mulder EJH, Mennes M *et al*. Antenatal maternal anxiety and stress and the neurobehavioural development of the fetus and child: links and possible mechanisms. A review. *Neuroscience and Biobehavioral Reviews* 2005; **29**: 237–58.

27 DiPietro JA, Costigan KA, Gurewitsch ED. Maternal psychophysiological change during the second half of gestation. *Biological Psychology* 2005; **69**: 23–38.

28 Field T, Hernandez-Reif M, Hart S *et al*. Pregnant women benefit from massage therapy. *Journal of Psychosomatic Obstetrics and Gynaecology* 1999; **20**: 31–8.

29 Field T, Diego M, Hernandez-Reif M *et al*. Pregnancy massage reduces prematurity, low birthweight and postpartum depression. *Infant Behavior and Development* 2009; **32**: 454–60.

30 Bosco Guerreiro da Silva J. Acupuncture for mild to moderate emotional complaints in pregnancy – a prospective, quasi-randomised, controlled study. *Acupuncture in Medicine* 2007; **25**: 65–71.

31 MacPherson H, Thomas K. Short-term reactions to acupuncture: a cross-sectional

survey of patient reports. *Acupuncture in Medicine* 2005; **23:** 112–20.

32 Johnson D. Acupuncture prior to and at embryo transfer in an assisted conception unit – a case series. *Acupuncture in Medicine* 2006; **24:** 23–8.

33 Stray-Pedersen B, Stray-Pedersen S. Etiologic factors and subsequent reproductive performance in 195 couples with a prior history of habitual abortion. *American Journal of Obstetrics and Gynecology* 1984; **148:** 140–46.

34 Brigham SA, Conlon C, Farquharson RG. A longitudinal study of pregnancy outcome following idiopathic recurrent miscarriage. *Human Reproduction* 1999; **14:** 2868–71.

35 Latendresse G. The interaction between chronic stress and pregnancy: preterm birth from a biobehavioral perspective. *Journal of Midwifery and Women's Health* 2009; **54:** 8–17.

36 Hogue CJR, Hoffman S, Hatch MC. Stress and preterm delivery: a conceptual framework. *Paediatric and Perinatal Epidemiology* 2001; **15 (Suppl. 2):** 30–40.

37 Elsenbruch S, Benson S, Rucke M *et al.* Social support during pregnancy: effects on maternal depressive symptoms, smoking and pregnancy outcome. *Human Reproduction* 2006; **22:** 869–77.

38 Love ER, Bhattacharya S, Smith NC *et al.* Effect of interpregnancy interval on outcomes of pregnancy after miscarriage: retrospective analysis of hospital episode statistics in Scotland. *BMJ* 2010; **341:** c3967.

39 Sood A, Ebbert JO, Sood R *et al.* Complementary treatments for tobacco cessation: a survey. *Nicotine and Tobacco Research* 2006; **8:** 767–71.

40 Franche RL. Psychologic and obstetric predictors of couples' grief during pregnancy after a miscarriage or perinatal death. *Obstetrics and Gynecology* 2001; **97:** 597–602.

41 Côté-Arsenault D, Donato KL, Earl SS. Watching and worrying: early pregnancy after loss experiences. *MCN American Journal of Maternal Child Nursing* 2006; **31:** 356–63.

42 Hill PD, DeBackere K, Kavanaugh KL. The parental experience of pregnancy after perinatal loss. *Journal of Obstetric, Gynecologic and Neonatal Nursing* 2008; **37:** 525–37.

43 Schott J, Henley A, Kohner N. *Pregnancy Loss and the Death of a Baby: guidelines for professionals.* 3rd edn. London: Sands; 2007.

FURTHER READING

- Field T. *Massage Therapy Research.* Edinburgh: Churchill Livingstone; 2006.
- Kastner J. *Chinese Nutrition Therapy.* Stuttgart: Thieme; 2004.
- Lewith G, Jonas WB, Walach H, eds. *Clinical Research in Complementary Therapies.* Edinburgh: Churchill Livingstone; 2002.
- Mills E, Duguoa J, Perri D *et al.* *Herbal Medicines in Pregnancy and Lactation.* London: Taylor & Francis; 2006.

- Peters D, ed. *Understanding the Placebo Effect in Complementary Medicine*. Edinburgh: Churchill Livingstone; 2001.
- Pitchford P. *Healing with Whole Foods*. 3rd edn. Berkeley, CA: North Atlantic Books; 2002.
- Pollan M. *In Defence of Food*. London: Allen Lane; 2008.

CHAPTER 8

Professional issues

INTRODUCTION

Working closely with couples who have lost a baby, irrespective of the gestational stage at which the loss occurred, can be an extremely challenging job for healthcare professionals. For medical staff working under great pressure and in demanding circumstances, the ability always to care compassionately for and support parents can sometimes be frustrated for reasons beyond their control, and this can lead to feelings of guilt and anxiety.[1] For practitioners working outside of mainstream healthcare, such as those in complementary and alternative medicine, without the structural support of an organisation to help to alleviate stress and offer opportunities for supportive discussion, the demands of working in this area of practice can be immense. This chapter discusses the importance of maintaining healthy patient–practitioner working relationships, and explores ways of avoiding professional burnout.

EMOTIONAL CHALLENGES FOR PRACTITIONERS

Providing professional care for women who have experienced pregnancy loss can be both highly stressful and extremely rewarding. Offering emotional space to allow women to describe the details of their experience requires an empathy and compassion that is vital for the therapeutic encounter to be successful. However, these discussions generate a variety of feelings in practitioners, and over time this has the potential to have an adverse emotional impact on them. While providing therapeutic support to women, practitioners also have to deal with their own feelings about the end of the pregnancy. This can be emotionally demanding in cases where the practitioner has been treating the patient for some time prior to conception. Feelings of professional failure and emotional attachment to the lost pregnancy can arise. For practitioners who are pregnant, or who may have lost a pregnancy themselves, the process of listening to their patients can sometimes provoke intensely personal responses.

The idea of the wounded healer

The idea of the 'wounded healer' dates back to ancient Greek mythology, according to which Chiron, wounded by the poisoned arrow of Heracles and destined to suffer endless pain, taught the healing arts to Asclepius, who became one of the founding fathers of Western medicine. Plato stated that the best physicians, rather than embodying perfect health themselves, were those who knew and experienced suffering themselves. The concept of the wounded healer has been exemplified in modern times by Carl Jung, with the therapeutic encounter between healer and patient having special potency if the healer has been wounded him- or herself. It is the idea that within each practitioner and each patient there is both a healer and patient, and it is through the stirring of the practitioner's own wounds that self-healing can be encouraged in the patient. According to Mitchell and Cormack,[2] the power of the therapeutic relationship between wounded healer and patient has three components.

1 The wounded healer may be able to activate the patient's own inner powers of recuperation by conveying a sense of the healer's own (symbolic) wound, which in turn will activate the patient's capacity to heal and thus contribute to self-healing. The wound of the practitioner should be implicit rather than explicit.

2 The wounded healer may be able to inspire the patient to recover and overcome their pain through example. In other words, if a patient knows that their practitioner has overcome difficulties, the practitioner can act as a coping role model and inspire confidence that the patient can do the same.

3 The wounded healer may be better able to understand the patient's experience and the patient's needs within the therapeutic relationship through their own suffering.

Clearly revelations that practitioners may be vulnerable have to be carefully managed, and must not lead to a state where the patient perceives the practitioner to be needy, or has a sense of having to take responsibility for the practitioner's well-being. There is a very clear distinction between those who have suffered enough to understand the pain of others and use it constructively, and those who have not recovered sufficiently and remain controlled by their experience. It is the process of recovery that contributes to the healing power of the wounded healer concept, not the wound itself. Practitioners who have not had direct experience of suffering or distress can still gain great insight into the subjective experiences of the women in their care by reading first-hand accounts[2] and support literature from groups such as the Miscarriage Association and the Stillbirth and Neonatal Death Society (SANDS), or the March of Dimes in the USA.

Burnout

Although a certain amount of stress is to be expected when working in an emotionally charged field, when stress becomes cumulative (*see* Box 8.1), extreme or exceeds an individual's ability to cope, burnout may result. Burnout syndrome is the exhaustion of the body's normal mechanisms for coping with stress. It can occur in those who work with people in a caring capacity, and is defined as a response to prolonged exposure to demanding interpersonal situations. It is characterised by emotional exhaustion, depersonalisation, and a reduced level of personal accomplishment.[3] In the context of practitioners, emotional exhaustion is said to occur when the practitioner is overwhelmed by their work, and is considered to be the first stage of burnout. Depersonalisation refers to impersonal feelings towards patients in one's care – that is, behaving as a carer but not feeling caring – and reduced personal accomplishment refers to the feeling that nothing that they do makes any difference, or that it remains unappreciated.

BOX 8.1: Common signs and symptoms of cumulative stress

Physical
- Overtiredness, diarrhoea, constipation, appetite changes, headaches, abdominal and back pains, sleep disturbances

Emotional
- Anxiety, frustration, guilt, mood swings, undue pessimism or optimism, irritability, apathy, resentment

Mental
- Forgetfulness, poor concentration, poor job performance, negative attitude, loss of creativity and motivation, boredom, negative self-talk, expectation of blame

Relational
- Feeling isolated, resentful or intolerant of others, loneliness, marriage problems, social withdrawal

Behavioural
- Increased intake of alcohol, taking up smoking, change in eating habits, hyperactivity, avoidance of situations, loss of sense of humour, cynicism

A high level of emotional involvement in their work without adequate social support or feelings of personal accomplishment may leave practitioners susceptible to burnout. Other factors that have been identified as contributing to burnout in doctors are the burden of administrative responsibilities, lack of autonomy, unclear rules and regulations, and excessive demands from managers and supervisors.[2] Although CAM practitioners tend to work autonomously, and therefore may be protected from some of the negative organisational pressures that are present in the NHS, for example, they do not have routine access to supportive networks and supervision.

Preventing burnout
The best way to prevent burnout is to promote personal and professional well-being at all levels. It is not always easy for practitioners to prioritise their own well-being until they become aware, through personal experience, of the problems that can occur when emotional health fails. Self-care is an essential tool that all practitioners should implement, and indeed they have a responsibility to do so, as only then will they be in sufficiently good emotional shape to care for their patients in a mutually positive relationship. It is an important mark of professional maturity and honesty when

practitioners recognise that they are fallible and vulnerable and they put in place measures to protect themselves. Steps that practitioners can take to prevent burnout include the following:

➤ *Start the day with a relaxing ritual.* Rather than getting straight out of bed in the morning, spend a few minutes meditating, doing gentle stretches, or reading something enjoyable.

➤ *Adopt healthy eating, exercising and sleeping habits.* Avoid faddy eating, skipping meals or overindulging. Recognise the need for sleep and adequate rest.

➤ *Set boundaries.* Learn to delegate or say 'no' to unwanted demands. If working from home, have set working hours, a separate work telephone, and times set aside when patients can have access to you.

➤ *Control your workload.*

➤ *Spend time with family and friends.* Protect family time and make it a priority. Make the effort to see friends regularly.

➤ *Take a regular break from technology.* Set a time each day when you completely disconnect. Stop checking your email, and switch off your phone and computer.

➤ *Release your creativity.* Try something new, or take up a hobby that you used to enjoy. Choose activities that have nothing to do with work, and do them regularly.

➤ *Learn how to manage stress.* Learning how to manage stress can help you to regain your balance (*see* Chapter 6).

➤ *Identify sources of personal and social support.* Network, and share ideas and problems with others. Ask for help when you need it.

➤ *Remain interested in new ideas.* Attending courses and conferences, reading professional literature, keeping up to date with knowledge, and discussing work with others all enhance one's resources. This is an aspect of self-care.

➤ *Adopt a healthy philosophical outlook on life and work.* Reassess what is important, and balance work with pleasure and relaxation. Bring joy and happy times back into your routine life. Take regular holidays and breaks from work.

➤ *Take up reflective activities.* This could be as varied as reading poetry, walking, swimming, spiritual practices, gardening, visiting art galleries, joining a book club, researching the family tree, and so on.

ETHICAL ISSUES
Ethical challenges for practitioners

Broadly speaking, ethics involves decisions and choices. Practitioners working with women who have experienced pregnancy loss may be challenged to act ethically themselves at all times, or find their own personal values challenged by the ethical dilemmas that are faced by their patients. The range of ethical issues that are raised by working in this field is endless, with some being relatively frequent and easily engaged with, while others are much less common (*see* Box 8.2). All health professions have their own ethical codes, but they are rarely specific, and there can be great challenges involved in applying them to practice. Certain healthcare professionals spend a lot of time with women, listening to and talking with them, and supporting and educating them. In the case of CAM practitioners, time is provided for women and their partners in a way that mainstream medicine can rarely allow, and as a result they will frequently reveal their own inner conflicts and dilemmas.

Much of CAM practice is centred on the importance of the practitioner–patient relationship, and the holistic and ongoing nature of this care can raise ethical issues that require special thought and consideration. It can be very frustrating, for example, if a pregnant woman is continuing to smoke or regularly drink alcohol despite a practitioner's best efforts to persuade her to change this behaviour. The practitioner may ask him- or herself why they should continue to treat the woman if she is failing to help herself, and whether it would be ethically reasonable to discontinue treatment in an attempt to persuade the woman to stop the harmful behaviour. Would this be abusing the influence of the practitioner–patient relationship, even if the intention behind the withdrawal from that relationship was morally sound? In terms of respecting patients' autonomy and their right to decide for themselves what is best, the ethical view may be that so long as the patient was informed and aware of the implications of her choices, her autonomy should be respected. However, in situations where the practitioner understands in detail the context of the patient's life, and the relationship is ongoing, the ethical position may be better viewed as one where this relationship is used to explore the obstacles to change that the patient is facing, and actions are then taken which bring about change. Healthcare professionals are most likely to face these types of issues when they have long-term contact with women, rather than when they are working in situations where they only see patients brief periods. CAM relationships are particularly likely to be of a long-term nature.

BOX 8.2: Examples of ethical challenges

- Previous history of termination
- Selective fetal reduction in multiple pregnancy
- Fetal reduction for abnormalities in multiple pregnancy
- Prenatal screening
- Termination of pregnancy on the grounds of congenital anomalies
- Assisted reproductive technologies
- Pre-implantation genetic diagnosis in IVF

It can be challenging if a patient undertakes a course of action or treatment with which the practitioner disagrees. For example, if the practitioner has personal objections to pregnancy termination, this might raise ethical challenges for them when treating a woman who decides to undergo selective fetal reduction. There is broad support in society for routine prenatal screening, which is in fact based on the assumption that in cases where serious fetal abnormalities are found, most parents will decide to have a termination.[4] However, until practitioners are faced with the reality of a patient undertaking this course of action, they may not realise the extent to which this may require them to examine their own personal values.

Virtue ethics

Broadly speaking, virtue ethics is Aristotelian in nature and links people's characters with their actions. Put simply, in virtue ethics a practitioner would reflect on their work by asking 'Am I doing the best thing for my patient?' rather than 'Is this ethical?'. The idea is that by nurturing ethical qualities or character traits, practitioners will act ethically. One problem with this approach is that there is no agreement on how such characteristics are developed in individuals. However, it does provide a useful practical framework for practitioners to think through their own ethical concerns. Corey *et al.*[5] have described five characteristics of virtuous professionals that form the core of virtue ethics:

➤ Practitioners are motivated to do the right thing because they judge it to be so, not because they feel obliged to do so, or because they fear the consequences.

➤ They rely on vision, discernment, understanding and sensitivity to reach judgements and take decisions.
➤ They have compassion, they are sensitive to the sufferings of people and they are able to take actions that reduce the pain of their patients.
➤ Virtuous practitioners are self-aware and know how their assumptions, values and biases will affect their interactions with those in their care.
➤ They are connected to their wider community and understand its ideals and expectations.

An example serves to illustrate how virtue ethics is helpful within the context of working with women who have experienced pregnancy loss. Suppose that a woman has a stillbirth and in her grief she decides that the best way for her to deal with the loss is to try to conceive again as soon as possible. She seeks treatment by an acupuncturist to help to improve her natural fertility and aid conception, and during the initial consultation she reveals that she has experienced bouts of depression throughout her life. During the course of the first few weeks of treatment it becomes clear to the practitioner that her patient is experiencing complicated grief. She is refusing to acknowledge or talk about the pregnancy and the death of her baby, she feels great anger towards her partner for not being ready to try to conceive again, and she says that she is refusing to see her wider family because she fears that they blame her for the loss. The practitioner knows that the woman requires more help than she is able to give her within the limits of her personal and professional competence. She has thought through questions of whether it would be ethical to continue to treat this patient in the knowledge that this was not offering her the best option for working through her grief. She has been wondering if by focussing on the woman's fertility, she was colluding in helping the patient to avoid the grief process. Would it be in the patient's best interest to stop seeing her for fertility support treatment in the hope that this would force her to address her grief? The practitioner also recognised that the patient had come to rely on the acupuncture sessions, and on her, and that on many levels the woman was benefiting from the treatment, so discontinuation of this could have a detrimental effect on her. After considering all aspects of the case, the practitioner decided that it was in the patient's best interest to seek bereavement counselling. Initially the patient was reluctant to accept this suggestion, as she was in denial of her grief. However, after she had heard the practitioner's caring explanations and acknowledgement of her own limitations, the woman did agree to be referred. She continued to receive acupuncture alongside the bereavement counselling.

Healthcare practitioners should be prepared to face difficult issues throughout their professional lives. Regularly thinking through their own values, beliefs and attitudes will enable them to focus on their patients' best interests, which is the most effective way to deal with ethical confusion and inner conflict.

REFERENCES

1 Schott J, Henley A, Kohner N. *Pregnancy Loss and the Death of a Baby: guidelines for professionals.* 3rd edn. London: Sands; 2007.

2 Mitchell A, Cormack M. *The Therapeutic Relationship in Complementary Health Care.* Edinburgh: Churchill Livingstone; 1998.

3 Maslach C, Jackson S, Leiter M. *Maslach Burnout Inventory Manual.* Palo Alto, CA: Consulting Psychologists Press; 1996.

4 Beeson D. *Social and Ethical Challenges of Prenatal Diagnosis.* www.lahey.org/PDF/Ethics/Winter_2000.pdf (accessed 3 September 2010).

5 Corey G, Schneider Corey M, Callanan P. *Issues and Ethics in the Helping Professions.* 7th edn. Belmont, CA: Thomson Higher Education; 2007.

FURTHER READING

- Cecil R, ed. *The Anthropology of Pregnancy Loss.* Oxford: Berg; 1996.
- Danielsson K. *After Miscarriage.* Boston, MA: Harvard Common Press; 2008.
- Moulder C. *Miscarriage: women's experiences and needs.* London: Routledge; 2001.

Resources and useful contacts

FAMILY, MULTIPLE BIRTHS AND BEREAVEMENT SUPPORT
Antenatal Results and Choices (ARC)
This is a national charity that provides non-directive support and information to expectant and bereaved parents throughout and after the antenatal screening and testing process.
73 Charlotte Street
London W1T 4PN
Tel: 0207 631 0280
Website: www.arc-uk.org

Baby Mailing Preference Service
This is a free service with which bereaved parents can register in order to reduce the number of baby-related mailings that they receive.
Freepost 29 LON20771
London W1E 0ZT
Tel: 0845 703 4599
Website: www.mpsonline.org.uk/bmpsr

Bliss
This charity offers support to premature and sick babies and their families.
9 Holyrood Street
London Bridge
London SE1 2EL
Tel: 020 7378 1122
Website: www.bliss.org.uk

Center for Loss in Multiple Birth (CLIMB)
This is an international support group for those who have experienced loss of a multiple birth.
Website: www.climb-support.org

Child Bereavement Charity
A charity that provides support, information and training to all families and professionals when a baby or child dies, or when a child is bereaved.
The Saunderton Estate
Wycombe Road
Saunderton
Buckinghamshire HP14 4BF
Tel: 01494 568900
Website: www.childbereavement.org.uk

The Compassionate Friends
This charity offers support and care from bereaved parents, siblings and grandparents for families who have suffered the death of a child/children.
53 North Street
Bristol BS3 1EN
Tel: 0845 120 3785
Website: www.tcf.org.uk

Cruse Bereavement Care
Tel: 0844 4779400
Website: www.crusebereavementcare.org.uk

Down's Syndrome Association
Tel: 0845 230 0372
Website: www.downs-syndrome.org.uk

March of Dimes
This US charity is dedicated to promoting the health of babies by preventing birth defects, premature birth, and infant mortality.
1275 Mamaroneck Avenue
White Plains
NY 10605
USA
Website: www.marchofdimes.com

Miscarriage Association
c/o Clayton Hospital
Northgate
Wakefield
West Yorkshire WF1 3JS
Tel: 01924 200799
Website: www.miscarriageassociation.org.uk

Multiple Births Foundation
Hammersmith House Level 4
Queen Charlotte's and Chelsea Hospital
Du Cane Road
London W12 0HS
Tel: 020 3313 3519
Website: www.multiplebirths.org.uk

Relate
This charity provides relationship support to couples and families.
Tel: 0300 1001234
Website: www.relate.org.uk

Stillbirth and Neonatal Death Society (SANDS)
28 Portland Place
London W1B 1LY
Tel: 020 7436 5881
Website: www.uk-sands.org

Twins and Multiple Births Association (TAMBA)
2 The Willows
Gardner Road
Guildford
Surrey GU1 4PG
Tel: 01483 304442
Website: www.tamba.org.uk

PREGNANCY SUPPORT AND INFORMATION
Association of Early Pregnancy Units
Website: www.earlypregnancy.org.uk

Early Pregnancy Group of the European Society of Human Reproduction and Embryology (ESHRE)
This group aims to provide a clinical and scientific link between the medical fields of infertility, human reproduction, prenatal diagnosis and fetal medicine.
Website: www.eshre.eu/01/default.aspx?pageid=61

National Childbirth Trust (NCT)
Tel: 0300 33 00 772
Website: www.nct.org.uk

HEALTH AND MEDICAL SUPPORT
Action on Pre-eclampsia
2c The Halfcroft
Syston LE7 1LD
Tel: 0116 2608088
Website: www.apec.org.uk

Action on Smoking and Health (ASH)
First Floor
144–145 Shoreditch High Street
London E1 6JE
Tel: 0207 739 5902
Website: www.ash.org.uk

Ectopic Pregnancy Trust
c/o 2nd Floor
Golden Jubilee Wing
King's College Hospital
Denmark Hill
London SE5 9RS
Tel: 020 7733 2653
Website: www.ectopic.org

Infertility Network UK
Charter House
43 St Leonards Road
Bexhill on Sea
East Sussex TN40 1JA
Tel: 0800 008 7464
Website: www.infertilitynetworkuk.com

QUIT
This charity aims to help smokers to stop smoking.
63 St Marys Axe
London EC3A 8AA
Tel: 0207 469 0400
Website: www.quit.org.uk

Verity: The PCOS Self-Help Group
New Bond House
124 New Bond Street
London W1S 1DX
Website: www.verity-pcos.org.uk

INFORMATION FOR HEALTHCARE PROFESSIONALS
National Center for Complementary and Alternative Medicine (NCCAM)
National Institutes of Health
9000 Rockville Pike
Bethesda
Maryland 20892
USA
Website: http://nccam.nih.gov

National Institute of Complementary Medicine (NICM)
Based in Australia, NICM was established to provide leadership and support for research into complementary medicine and translation of evidence into clinical practice.
Website: http://nicm.edu.au

Perinatal Institute for Maternal and Child Health
The Perinatal Institute's primary focus is on understanding the causes and developing strategies for the prevention of perinatal compromise.
Crystal Court
Aston Cross
Birmingham B6 5RQ
Tel: 0121 687 3400
Website: www.perinatal.nhs.uk

International Stillbirth Alliance (ISA)
This non-profit coalition of organisations is dedicated to understanding the causes and prevention of stillbirth.
1314 Bedford Avenue, Suite 210
Baltimore
MD 21208
USA
Website: www.stillbirthalliance.org

UK GOVERNMENT HEALTH REGULATORY ORGANISATIONS
Food Standards Agency
Tel: 020 7276 8829
Website: www.food.gov.uk

Human Fertilisation and Embryology Authority
21 Bloomsbury Street
London WC1B 3HF
Tel: 0207 291 8200
Website: www.hfea.gov.uk

PRACTITIONER ORGANISATIONS AND INFORMATION
British Acupuncture Council
63 Jeddo Road
London W12 9HQ
Tel: 0208 7350400
Website: www.acupuncture.org

British Medical Acupuncture Society (BMAS)
Royal London Hospital for Integrated Medicine (formerly Royal London Homoeopathic Hospital)
60 Great Ormond Street
London WC1N 3HR
Tel: 020 7713 9437
Website: www.medical-acupuncture.co.uk

International Federation of Professional Aromatherapists (IFPA)
82 Ashby Road
Hinckley
Leicestershire LE10 1SN
Tel: 01455 637987
Website: www.ifparoma.org

British Association for Counselling and Psychotherapy (BACP)
15 St John's Business Park
Lutterworth LE17 4HB
Tel: 01455 883300
Website: www.bacp.co.uk

National Institute of Medical Herbalists (NIMH)
Elm House
54 Mary Arches Street
Exeter EX4 3BA
Tel: 01392 426022
Website: www.nimh.org.uk

Register of Chinese Herbal Medicine (RCHM)
Office 5
1 Exeter Street
Norwich NR2 4QB
Tel: 01603 623994
Website: www.rchm.co.uk

Society of Homeopaths
11 Brookfield, Duncan Close
Moulton Park
Northampton NN3 6WL
Tel: 0845 450 6611
Website: www.homeopathy-soh.org

British Society of Clinical Hypnosis
125 Queensgate
Bridlington
East Yorkshire YO16 7JQ
Tel: 01262 403103
Website: www.bsch.org.uk

British Association for Applied Nutrition and Nutritional Therapy
27 Old Gloucester Street
London WC1N 3XX
Tel: 08706 061284
Website: www.bant.org.uk

Royal College of Obstetricians and Gynaecologists (RCOG)
27 Sussex Place
Regent's Park
London NW1 4RG
Tel: 020 7772 6200
Website: www.rcog.org.uk

Association of Reflexologists (AoR)
5 Fore Street
Taunton
Somerset TA1 1HX
Tel: 01823 351010
Website: www.aor.org.uk

International Federation of Reflexologists (IFR)
8–9 Talbot Court
London EC3V 0BP
Tel: 0870 879 3562
Website: www.intfedreflexologists.org

Yoga Biomedical Trust
31 Dagmar Road
London N22 7RT
Tel: 020 8245 6420
Website: www.yogatherapy.org

British Wheel of Yoga
25 Jermyn Street
Sleaford
Lincolnshire NG34 7RU
Tel: 01529 306851
Website: www.bwy.org.uk

Index